THE
KIDNEY

ATLAS *of* TUMOR RADIOLOGY

PHILIP J. HODES, M.D., *Editor-in-Chief*

Sponsored by

THE AMERICAN COLLEGE OF RADIOLOGY

—*with the cooperation of:*

AMERICAN CANCER SOCIETY
AMERICAN ROENTGEN RAY SOCIETY
CANCER CONTROL PROGRAM, USPHS
EASTMAN KODAK COMPANY
JAMES PICKER FOUNDATION
RADIOLOGICAL SOCIETY OF NORTH AMERICA

THE
KIDNEY

by

JOHN A. EVANS, M.D.

Professor and Chairman of the Department of Radiology,
Cornell University Medical College,
and Radiologist-in-Chief to The New York Hospital

and

MORTON A. BOSNIAK, M.D.

Professor of Radiology, New York University School of Medicine,
and Chief, Section of Uroradiology,
New York University Medical Center

YEAR BOOK MEDICAL PUBLISHERS · INC.

35 EAST WACKER DRIVE, CHICAGO

Dedicated to

DOROTHY, LINDA, JANE, JOHN *and* SUSAN
and to LINDIE

Editor's Preface

In 1960, the Committee on Radiology of the National Research Council began to consider the preparation of a tumor atlas for radiology similar in concept to the Armed Forces Institute of Pathology's "Atlas of Tumor Pathology." So successfully had the latter filled a need in pathology that it seemed reasonable to establish a similar resource for radiology. Therefore a subcommittee of the Committee on Radiology was appointed to study the concept and make recommendations.

That original committee, made up of Dr. Russell H. Morgan (Chairman), Dr. Marshall H. Brucer and Dr. Eugene P. Pendergrass, reported that a need did indeed exist and recommended that something be done about it. That report was unanimously accepted by the parent committee.

Soon thereafter, there occurred a normal change of the membership of the Committee on Radiology of the Council. This was followed by a change of the "Atlas" subcommittee, which now included Dr. E. Richard King (Chairman), Dr. Leo G. Rigler and Dr. Barton R. Young. To this new subcommittee was assigned the task of finding how the "Atlas" was to be published. Numerous avenues were explored; none seemed wholly satisfactory.

With the passing of time, it became increasingly apparent that the American College of Radiology had to be brought into the picture. It had prime teaching responsibilities; it had a Commission on Education; it seemed the logical responsible agent to launch the "Atlas." Confident of the merits of this approach, the entire Committee on Radiology of the Council became involved in focusing the attention of the American College of Radiology upon the matter.* In 1964, as the result of their persuasiveness, the Board of Chancellors of the American College of Radiology named an ad hoc committee to explore and define the scholarly scope of the "Atlas" and the probable costs. In 1965, the ad hoc committee recommended that the College sponsor and publish the "Atlas." Accordingly, an Editorial Advisory Com-

---

* At that time, the Committee on Radiology included, in addition to the subcommittee, Drs. John A. Campbell, James B. Dealy, Jr., Melvin M. Figley, Hymer L. Friedell, Howard B. Latourette, Alexander Margulis, Ernest A. Mendelsohn, Charles M. Nice, Jr., and Edward W. Webster.

mittee was chosen to work within the Commission on Education with authority to select an Editor-in-Chief. At the same time, the College provided funds for starting the project and began representations for grants-in-aid without which the "Atlas" would never be published.

No history of the "Atlas of Tumor Radiology" would be complete without specific recording of the generous response of the several radiological societies, as well as the private and Federal granting institutions whose names appear on the title page and below among our acknowledgments. It was their tangible evidence of confidence in the project that provided everyone with enthusiasm and eagerness to achieve our goal.

The "Atlas of Tumor Radiology" includes all major organ systems. It is intended to be a systematic body of pictorial and written information dealing with the roentgen manifestations of tumors. No attempt has been made to provide an atlas equivalent of a medical encyclopedia. Nevertheless the "Atlas" is designed to serve as an important reference source and teaching file for all physicians, not radiologists alone.

The thirteen volumes of the "Atlas," to be completed in 1971–72, are: *The Hemopoietic and Lymphatic Systems,* by Gerald D. Dodd and Sidney Wallace; *The Bones and Joints,* by Gwilym S. Lodwick (published); *The Chest,* by Roy R. Greening and J. Haynes Heslep; *The Gastrointestinal Tract,* by Arthur K. Finkelstein and George N. Stein; *The Kidney,* by John A. Evans and Morton A. Bosniak (published); *The Lower Urinary Tract, Adrenals and Retroperitoneum,* by Morton A. Bosniak, Stanley S. Siegelman and John A. Evans; *The Breast,* by David M. Witten (published); *The Head and Neck,* by Gilbert H. Fletcher and Bao-Shan Jing (published); *The Brain and Eye,* by Ernest W. Wood, Juan M. Taveras and Michael S. Tenner; *The Female Reproductive System,* by G. Melvin Stevens (published); *The Endocrines,* by Howard L. Steinbach and Hideyo Minagi (published); *The Accessory Digestive Organs,* by Robert F. Wise and Augustine P. O'Keeffe; and *The Spine,* by Bernard S. Epstein.

Some overlapping of material in several volumes is inevitable, for example, tumors of the female generative system, tumors of the endocrine glands and tumors of the urinary tract. This is considered to be an asset. It assures the specialist completeness in the volume or volumes that concern him and provides added breadth and depth of knowledge for those interested in the entire series.

The broad scope of the "Atlas of Tumor Radiology" has precluded its preparation by a single or even several authors. To maintain uniformity of format, rather rigid criteria were established early. These included manner of presentation, size of illustrations, as well as style of headings, subheadings and legends. The authors were encouraged to keep the text at a minimum, freeing as much space as possible for large illustrations and meaningful legends. The "Atlas" is to be just that, an "atlas," not a series of "texts." The authors were urged, also, to keep the bibliography brief.

The selection of suitable authors for the "Atlas" was extremely difficult, and to a degree invidious. For the final choice, the Editor-in-Chief accepts full responsibility. It is but fair to record, however, that his Editorial Advisory Committee accepted his recommendations. The format of the "Atlas," too, was the choice of the Editor-in-Chief, again with the concurrence of his advisory group. Should the "Atlas of Tumor Radiology" fall short of its goals, the fault will lie with the Editor-in-Chief alone; his Editorial Advisory Committee was selfless in its dedication to the purposes of the "Atlas," rendering invaluable advice and guidance whenever asked to do so.

As medical knowledge expands, medical concepts change. In medicine, the written word considered true today may not be so tomorrow. The text of the "Atlas," considered true today, therefore may not be true tomorrow. What may not change, what may ever remain true, may be the illustrations of the "Atlas of Tumor Radiology." Their legends may change as our conceptual levels advance. But the validity of the roentgen findings there recorded should endure. Thus, if the fidelity with which the roentgenograms have been reproduced is of superior order, the illustrations in the "Atlas" should long serve as sources for reference no matter what revisions of the text become necessary with advancing medical knowledge.

ACKNOWLEDGMENTS

The American College of Radiology, its Commission on Education, the Editorial Advisory Committee, the authors and the Editor-in-Chief wish to acknowledge their grateful appreciation:

1. For the grants-in-aid so willingly and repeatedly provided by The American Cancer Society, The American Roentgen Ray Society, The Cancer Control Program, National Center for Chronic Disease Control (USPHS Grant No. 59481), The James Picker Foundation, and The Radiological Society of North America.

2. For the superb glossy print reproductions provided by the Radiography Markets Division, Eastman Kodak Company. Special mention must be made of the sustained interest of Mr. George R. Struck, its Assistant Vice-President and General Manager. We applaud particularly Mr. William S. Cornwell, Technical Associate and Editor Emeritus of Kodak's *Medical*

Radiography and Photography, as well as his associates, Mr. Charles C. Heckman and Mr. David Edwards and others in the Photo Service Division, whose expertise provided the "Atlas" with its incomparable photographic reproductions.

3. To Year Book Medical Publishers, for their personal involvement with and judicious guidance in the many problems of publication. There were occasions when the publisher questioned the quality of certain illustrations. Almost always the judgment of the authors and the Editor-in-Chief prevailed because of the importance of the original roentgenograms and the singular fidelity of their reproduction.

4. To the Associate Editors, particularly Mrs. Anabel I. Janssen, whose talents lightened the burden of the Editor-in-Chief and helped establish the style of presentation of the material.

5. To the Staff of the American College of Radiology, especially Messrs. William C. Stronach, Otha Linton, Keith Gundlach and William Melton, for continued conceptual and administrative efforts of unusual competence.

This volume has brought together two important contributors to our knowledge concerning the radiologic aspects of diseases of the urinary tract. It represents not the simple summation of the experiences of two acknowledged authorities in the field. Instead, we find one author stimulating the other, sharpening insight and heightening communication to their mutual benefit and thus to the benefit of this volume of the "Atlas." The work is a fortunate blending of the recent past and the present which tends to foretell the future. The interested student will find here carefully selected books of knowledge, fused logically, upon which he may build securely.

Originally this volume of the "Atlas" was to include not only the kidney but the ureter, adrenals, bladder and their intimate neighboring structures. As work progressed it became obvious that such a volume would be too large for the reader to handle with ease. It was decided, therefore, to split it into two volumes, the first dealing with the kidneys themselves and the second with the rest of the urinary tract—the ureters, adrenals, bladder and retroperitoneal structures. The latter volume should be available within a year.

As one thumbs through the pages of this volume, one is impressed by the wide range of techniques available and essential for the diagnosis of renal disease. The body harbors no other organ in behalf of which more varied radiographic procedures are available for diagnosis. They run the gamut from simple radiographic exposures to the most complex and selective form of pharmacoradiology. With the best interests of the patient in mind. the hope is that no more exposure to radiation will be used than is essential to establish a diagnosis. This is not to deny the importance, and indeed absolute need, for developing new knowledge. It is to say, however, that studied judgment and keen appreciation of routine roentgen findings may render additional studies unnecessary when casual investigation or a desire for perfectionism might suggest them.

The "Atlas of Tumor Radiology" is being published at a time when massive scientific effort is taking place at an unprecedented rate and on an unprecedented scale. We hope that our final product will provide an authoritative summary of our current knowledge of the roentgen manifestations of tumors.

PHILIP J. HODES
Editor-in-Chief

New Jersey College of Medicine and Dentistry
Newark, New Jersey

Editorial Advisory Committee

HARRY L. BERMAN   VINCENT P. COLLINS   E. RICHARD KING
LEO G. RIGLER   PHILIP RUBIN

Authors' Preface

DIAGNOSTIC RADIOLOGY provides a graphic method of demonstrating renal tumor pathology. Technical advances in the recent past have greatly enhanced the detection, demonstration and diagnosis of renal tumors. In particular, the use of angiography enables the radiologist to define clearly the nature and extent of renal tumor pathology prior to surgery or necropsy. Extension of tumor into the retroperitoneal space, into the vena cava or to adjacent or distant organs can be demonstrated accurately by angiographic techniques. On occasion, angiography can even be used as a substitute for a histopathologic biopsy in the evaluation of a patient with renal carcinoma.

The improved ability to detect and diagnose renal tumors is of considerable importance in deciding the proper treatment for a patient with a renal mass. Radiology can establish whether a mass is a cyst or tumor and as a result has saved countless numbers of needless explorations for benign disease. Furthermore, nephrectomy is simplified by the preoperative demonstration of the nature and extent of the pathology and the vascular anatomy.

We have tried to demonstrate the full range of the radiographic presentations of renal carcinoma. Its varied appearances and manifestations are depicted. The difficulties in diagnosing hypovascular tumors have been emphasized by the inclusion of many such examples.

A small section on cystic disease is included. This is a far from complete presentation of this complex subject and its purpose is to illustrate the differential diagnostic aspects of cystic disease and neoplastic disease in the context of the diagnosis of a renal mass. A section on pseudoneoplasms of the kidney is also presented to emphasize that a number of non-neoplastic conditions (besides cystic disease) can be mistaken for renal neoplasms and must be considered in the radiographic evaluation of renal mass lesions.

While a major portion of the book is devoted to renal cell carcinoma and its varied manifestations, the other more common renal tumors such as renal pelvic tumors, Wilms' tumor and metastatic tumor are also dealt with in some detail. Although we have attempted to show an example of as many of the rare renal neoplasms as possible, we have not been able to include every possible type of renal lesion that has been reported. This would be an almost endless task and in our opinion of limited value, as the radiologic diagnosis for most of them is not specific even though their histologic characteristics may be.

The amount of written text and references has been kept to a minimum, as is the policy of the "Atlas," with maximum information to be derived from the illustrations and their descriptions, and appropriate comments. We have included a number of recent and more important references on some of the material presented so that the reader will have a starting point if he wants to search the literature for further information. We know that we have omitted a number of important references and hope that our colleagues who have authored them will forgive us.

It is beyond the capabilities of one or two authors and beyond the resources of one or two institutions to assemble the variety of kidney tumor pathology contained in this volume. This could only be accomplished through the cooperation of many radiologists who were generous with their material and made it available to us. Acknowledgment to these radiologists appears with the case that they have contributed; we are grateful for being permitted to use this case material.

The great bulk of material, however, was gleaned from our own experiences at the hospitals at which we have served—Dr. Evans at The New York Hospital-Cornell Medical Center and Dr. Bosniak, who has been associated with a number of institutions including Montefiore Hospital and Medical Center, Boston University Medical Center, Albert Einstein College Hospital and the New York University Medical Center. At these institutions we have worked closely with our colleagues in the performance and/or interpretation of most of these cases. We would like to express our thanks to all of those radiologists and urologists who have worked with us over the past years. Particular thanks are extended to Dr. Robin Watson of The New York Hospital-Cornell Medical Center, the late Dr. Saul (Whitey) Scheff of Boston University Medical Center, Dr. Robert Bernstein of Albert Einstein College Hospital and Dr. Manuel Madayag of New York University Medical Center.

We also thank our secretaries, who were of great help to us throughout this work—Miss Julia Mala, Mrs. Eve Ponzio and Mrs. Mary Ann Prudenti.

Last, we acknowledge with gratitude the help, advice and understanding of our Editor-in-Chief, Dr. Philip J. Hodes, for his unwavering faith in the eventuality of this text.

JOHN A. EVANS
MORTON A. BOSNIAK

PART 1

Radiographic Techniques of Examination of the Urinary Tract

Radiographic Techniques of Examination

RADIOLOGICALLY, the urinary tract is one of the most readily accessible systems in the body and numerous techniques have been developed to study it. Some have been available for many years and their role in diagnostic radiology has been well established; others are of more recent development and the full significance of their contribution has not been completely realized. A review of these techniques follows, with a discussion of the relative importance of each, their reliability and the role of each in the study of a patient with a renal tumor.

INTRAVENOUS UROGRAPHY

Intravenous urography is the basic screening procedure for study of the urinary tract, retroperitoneal space and adrenal glands. It determines kidney function, position and structure and outlines the character and anatomy of the collecting systems. Information that can be obtained from this study has a wide range of specificity. In some instances, a definitive diagnosis is obtained and no further radiologic workup is required; for example, pelvic kidney or medullary sponge kidney. On the other hand, the urogram may disclose an abnormality that requires further radiographic examination for definitive diagnosis, as in the case of a renal mass.

Intravenous urography was introduced for medical diagnosis by von Lichtenberg and Swick in 1929. Since then there has been continuous improvement in the quality and safety of the contrast mediums used. The introduction of newer, safer contrast agents has significantly enhanced the diagnostic value of the intravenous urogram and has permitted the use of larger volumes in routine studies. Drip infusion techniques combined with tomography provide excellent delineation of the renal parenchyma and collecting system. Delineation of renal parenchyma and the collecting system has greatly enhanced the accuracy of diagnosis of urinary tract disease particularly with respect to the detection of renal mass lesions.

RETROGRADE PYELOGRAPHY

Prior to the development of intravenous pyelography, retrograde pyelography was the only method available for demonstrating intrarenal structure. At present, its use is limited to a few specific conditions. These include the obtaining of information about renal morphology when this cannot be done by intravenous urography. Its most generally accepted indication is the detection and localization of lesions involving the pelvicalyceal system and ureter; for this purpose it is not only valuable but frequently essential. Retrograde pyelography provides little in the study of diseases involving the renal parenchyma, particularly tumors. Nor is it ordinarily useful in the problem of extrarenal masses. It may be helpful in certain cases of unexplained hematuria, when excretory urography and cystoscopy reveal no abnormalties. Its use is indicated in evaluating the cause of a nonvisualized kidney on intravenous urography. The differentiation of a huge neoplasm with renal vein obstruction, a hydronephrotic sac and a multicystic kidney (all of which would present as masses with nonvisualization on intravenous urography) can be made by retrograde study. This differentiation can also be made by other modalities (renal arteriography) in certain instances when retrograde pyelography is contraindicated or cannot be performed.

RETROPERITONEAL GAS INSUFFLATION

This technique has limited value in the diagnosis of renal and retroperitoneal tumors and has largely been supplanted by nephrotomography and renal arteriography. The technique is performed by the injection of 500–1000 cc of carbon dioxide (or nitrous oxide) into the retroperitoneal space via either the presacral or the perirenal approach. It is used mainly to outline the structures in the retroperitoneal space, to differentiate renal from extrarenal neoplasms and to visualize the adrenal glands. An inability to differentiate cyst from neoplasm limits its usefulness in renal disease. Its primary application is in the detection of adrenal tumors, and when used for this purpose the diagnostic value can be enhanced by combining it with tomography or nephrotomography. The introduction of adrenal angiography and selective adrenal venography limits even further the use of retroperitoneal air insufflation.

NEPHROTOMOGRAPHY

Nephrotomography is a relatively simple, inexpensive radiographic examination that can be performed with a minimum of experience and equipment. It is associated with a high diagnostic yield particularly in the differentiation of renal cyst and neoplasm. It also is of considerable importance in differentiating renal from extrarenal neoplasms and in demonstrating the size and shape of the adrenal glands.

The technique originally described by Evans *et al.* and later modified by

Shenker is basically the performance of tomography of the kidneys during the nephrogram phase that occurs following the rapid introduction of a large quantity of concentrated contrast agent intravenously. In the more recently adapted drip infusion technique, 125 cc of a concentrated urographic medium (90% Hypaque) in 75 cc glucose and water is delivered intravenously through an 18 gauge needle as fast as possible. Tomograms of the kidneys are taken after one-half of the contrast has been delivered and while the remainder of the solution is being injected. "Tomographic cuts" are taken at multiple levels (6–11 cm for average size patients). Films are then taken in anteroposterior position of both kidneys and the appropriate oblique position (right posterior oblique for the right kidney, left posterior oblique for the left kidney). Great care in radiographic detail is essential if this technique is to achieve its full potential. Proper coning, precise radiographic technique and adequate speed of injection of contrast medium are absolutely critical if a high degree of accuracy is to be obtained.

The primary *advantages* of nephrotomography are: (1) Has use as a further screening procedure in cases that are questionable on intravenous urography; for example, bulge in the kidney contour. (2) Differentiates renal cyst from solid tumor of the cortex. (3) Helps in differentiating extrarenal from renal masses. (4) Delineates the adrenal gland. (5) Enables more complete filling and visualization of the collecting system. (6) Has a value in studying elderly arteriosclerotic patients in whom renal arteriography may present an increased risk. (7) Is easy and inexpensive to perform and can be done on outpatients.

Limitations of the method include: (1) Its limited value in patients with chronic renal disease in whom adequate nephrograms cannot be obtained. (2) Whereas the method permits a conclusive diagnosis of either cyst or neoplasm as a rule, there are individuals in whom the differentiation is not clearly defined. (3) It cannot be used alone to make a definitive diagnosis in lesions that are totally intrarenal (see Fig. 4).

When the nephrotomographic criteria for a simple cyst are totally fulfilled, as described in Figures 3, 5 and 6, the accuracy of nephrotomography alone may approach 100%. However, if *all the criteria* are not totally fulfilled, a diagnosis of simple cyst cannot be made on the basis of nephrotomography alone. In the latter eventuality, arteriography must be performed.

Nephrotomography should not be considered to be in competition with arteriography, but rather, should be used as a supplementary procedure. This is particularly true in the study of difficult renal lesions. Some are best identified by nephrotomography, others by arteriography. By combining the two techniques, a diagnostic accuracy approaching 100% may be realized.

Aortography was first performed by Dos Santos Lamas in 1929 via a translumbar needle injection into the abdominal aorta. This technique was subsequently used primarily to study occlusive disease of the aorta, its branches and the peripheral circulation. Although capable of providing useful information about the renal vasculature and parenchyma, it had limited value because of several major disadvantages. These included: (1) The use of general anesthesia; (2) restricted mobility of the patient; (3) difficulty in utilizing rapid serial film equipment, and (4) significant incidence of serious complications.

It was not until the introduction of the Seldinger catheter technique of arteriography, the utilization of rapid serial film changers (and other related technical advances—image intensification, etc.), the introduction of safer contrast agents and the widespread use of selective renal catheterization that renal angiography developed into one of the most accurate diagnostic methods available in clinical medicine.

Renal arteriography is generally recognized as the single most valuable radiologic means for studying the renal vessels and the renal parenchyma. To achieve maximal diagnostic results the technique requires an examination routine that allows a complete angiographic evaluation of the patient's renal status. This routine should include: (1) A preliminary or survey type "flush" aortogram (midstream aortic injection). The basic aortogram will provide essential information about the character of the blood supply to both kidneys. Frequently this is adequate to make a definitive diagnosis and no further examination is necessary. (2) Selective angiography of the appropriate vessels. This may provide further diagnostic information or may in fact be essential to the diagnosis in many cases.

In approximately 75% of cases of renal carcinoma, the diagnosis of malignancy can be made by the flush aortogram itself since the tumor vasculature is sufficiently abundant and obvious to be detected by this procedure. About 20% of the lesions can be detected only if selective angiography is performed since the tumor vasculature is sparse and can be visualized only with more selective method. Five per cent of the lesions have no demonstrable "tumora vessels" and are considered "avascular." However, these lesions can be diagnosed correctly by the use of supplement procedures (nephrotomography, epinephrine angiography, magnification, etc.) and interpretative experience. Clinical experience, technical skill, proper equipment and a carefully followed radiographic plan of study are the ingredients necessary for diagnostic success.

Renal arteriography, in addition to its diagnostic value, provides important anatomic information for the surgeon. The number, size and position of renal arteries, the total vascular supply of a renal tumor and evidence of extracapsular extension of tumor, renal vein invasion or metastases to other organs or tissues are examples of anatomic information that can decisively influence the surgical management of a patient. The diagnosis of a malignant renal neoplasm permits the urologic surgeon to proceed immediately to a radical nephrectomy without the need of first performing a renal biopsy. The arteriographic demonstration of metastatic disease could result in the decision to use radiation or chemotheraphy or both in lieu of surgery as the primary means of treatment.

PHARMACOLOGIC ANGIOGRAPHY.—The use of pharmacologic agents at the time of renal angiography has proved helpful in certain problem cases.

The drug most commonly used and the one with which most experience has been accumulated is epinephrine. Epinephrine, a potent vasoconstrictor, was shown by Abrams to have less effect on "tumor vessels" than on normal renal vasculature. Therefore if, just prior to angiography, epinephrine is administered intrarenally (through the selective renal artery catheter), the resultant angiogram is more sensitive in detecting a malignant lesion because the normal vessels are constricted and poorly visualized while the tumor vessels are less affected and therefore better visualized. Potentially, this technique can bring out the abnormal vascularity of hypovascular or "avascular" renal neoplasms. We have seen two instances in which a conventional study failed to reveal a renal malignancy which was then appreciated with the use of epinephrine angiography. The technique also has value in lesions that are questionable on conventional angiography (Figs. 42 and 43). A "positive epinephrine test" will more clearly establish a malignant lesion while a negative test will prove more conclusively that the lesion is benign. We have seen a number of confusing benign conditions (particularly renal columns projecting into the renal sinus) in which malignancy could effectively be ruled out with the use of the epinephrine technique.

Briefly, the procedure is performed by injecting 5–10 µg of epinephrine (diluted to a 10 ml solution) intrarenally through the selective renal catheter 10 seconds prior to angiography. Filming is then performed over a 20 second period (1/second) as the renal flow is slowed. Experience is necessary to get maximal information from the test, because dose and timing can be critical.

Epinephrine is also used in the study of adrenal arteries and renal veins, as described on page 11. The use of this drug has definitely found a place in the study of renal neoplasms and its use by angiographers is encouraged to enhance further the diagnostic accuracy of renal angiography.

A number of other drugs, mainly vasodilators, have also been used in renal angiography both clinically and experimentally to improve delineation of renal vascular structures. So far these have had limited success. Clearly, further work along these lines is needed before we can be certain of their ultimate value.

MAGNIFICATION ANGIOGRAPHY.—A further addition to the technology of renal angiography in the evaluation of renal tumors has been the development of radiographic magnification. The technique requires the use of a special fine focal spot tube (0.3 mm or less) with radiographic magnification achieved by increasing the object–film distance.

With the use of this technique, 2–3 times magnification is obtained which will enhance the visualization of smaller vessels not fully appreciated by conventional means. The potential of this technique is that hypovascular or so-called avascular malignant lesions will be better studied and less likely to escape detection. In our experience, the technique has indeed improved the demonstration of abnormal vessels associated with hypovascular lesions (Fig. 45). Although it does bring out these vessels somewhat more strikingly, we have not encountered a case in which a diagnosis could be made with magnification techniques that could not be appreciated with conventional angiography. However, the potential value of the method is appreciated and further experience with its use is clearly indicated.

CYST PUNCTURE AND OPACIFICATION

Percutaneous cyst puncture as a diagnostic technique for the differentiation of cyst from tumor was first described by Fish in 1939. Cyst puncture is simplified by prior opacification of the kidney and the use of television fluoroscopy. Large lower pole masses lend themselves readily to cyst puncture. Fluid is aspirated (for cytologic examination) and replaced by contrast medium, followed by radiography of the contrast-filled cavity in various projections in order to study the entire circumference of the cyst wall. A smooth sharp margin is seen in a benign cyst, whereas irregularity of the wall suggests malignancy. Double-contrast opacification studies have also been used, with the injection of air as well as radiopaque contrast agents to enhance evaluation of the cyst wall. Proponents of this technique feel that it is the only method short of surgery that will exclude a small carcinoma growing in the wall of a cyst (see Fig. 60). This group advocates the use of cyst puncture as a further proof in all patients in whom surgical exploration is not planned.

Therapeutic cyst puncture with the instillation of Pantopaque was recommended by Vestby. The oily contrast agent provokes a foreign body reaction that stimulates permanent shrinkage of the cyst.

The role of cyst puncture and opacification, however, has not been generally accepted. There is differing opinion as to the necessity and safety of the procedure. Opponents feel that the possibility of dissemination of tumor cells, if a malignancy is encountered, does not justify this approach. They argue that if there is any doubt as to the identity of a renal mass lesion, exploratory surgery should be performed. Cyst puncture, however, would seem to be useful in poor-risk patients in whom a clearcut diagnosis of benign cyst is not possible by nephrotomography or angiography.

NEPHROSONOGRAPHY

The use of ultrasound has added a new dimension to the diagnosis of renal masses. The technique is based on the differences in the amount of reflected waves or echoes which occur between solid and fluid tissues as well as at interfaces between tissues. A cystic mass will give a maximal reflection due to the fluid–solid interface found in these lesions, whereas a solid tumor will produce a weaker echo complex since a solid–solid interface is present. Analysis of the tracing obtained can therefore be expected to differentiate these lesions. In over 100 cases, Goldberg *et al.* claimed an accuracy of 95%. The method is simple, inexpensive and nontraumatic. Further experience with the procedure will, of course, be necessary before it is assigned a definite place in the evaluation of renal mass lesions. The technique adds no further accuracy in detecting the difficult-to-diagnose cystic carcinomas. Nor does it furnish the valuable anatomic information provided by the angiographic techniques. Its major value seems to be as a supplement to nephrotomography or arteriography or both. However, it may well have specific indications, as in the case of old debilitated patients and those sensitive to contrast agents. The development of more sensitive instrumentation may improve its diagnostic accuracy and extend its range of usefulness. At the time of writing we feel that the technique should be used not as a definitive means of diagnosing renal masses but only as a supplement to corroborate findings obtained by nephrotomography or renal angiography.

ISOTOPES (RADIONUCLIDES)

In recent years there has been considerable enthusiasm for the use of radionuclides to study various organs and neoplasms. These techniques have been successful and enjoy widespread use in the study of neoplasms of the brain and liver but have been less useful in other organs. Some work has been done in the study of neoplasms of the kidney, but the value of isotope procedures for this purpose is still questionable. Further refinements in instrumentation and development of more specific radionuclides may increase the importance of isotope scanning techniques in the diagnosis of renal masses.

The differentiation of renal cyst from tumor is based on the following points. If chlormerodrin (^{197}Hg) is given intravenously, it will be picked up by the tubular cells of the kidney. A defect in the scan suggests an area devoid of functioning tubular mass which could be either cyst or tumor. Now, however, if an intravenous injection of sodium pertechnetate (^{99m}Tc) is made, the vascularity of the lesion can be studied. According to Rosenthall, an avascular lesion would presumably represent a benign cyst, and vascularity in the lesion would indicate malignancy. As a screening procedure, the technique has some merit but cannot be considered a definitive method for the study of renal mass lesions.

Inferior Venacavography; Renal Phlebography

Opacification of the inferior vena cava is a simple but extremely informative technique for evaluating retroperitoneal tumors and for determining the presence and the extent of venous invasion by a renal malignancy.

The examination is performed either by bilateral needle punctures of the femoral veins or by passage of a catheter percutaneously (via a femoral vein) into the distal inferior vena cava. Following the injection of contrast medium, films are obtained in the anteroposterior and lateral (or steep right posterior oblique) projections. The position, patency and integrity of the inferior vena cava can be then ascertained.

Inferior venacavography should be performed in all cases of renal carcinoma. Kidney carcinoma commonly invades the renal vein and may extend into the inferior vena cava and sometimes even into the right atrium. Preoperative knowledge of the extent of venous involvement aids the surgeon in careful planning of the operative attack. Also, prognosis is clarified by demonstration of the extent of spread of the neoplasm.

Selective renal phlebography can be done if the cavogram reveals the inferior vena cava to be free from tumor. Selective catheterization of the renal veins carries with it the risk of dislodging tumor thrombus and thus is not without hazard. Furthermore, the same information obtained from renal phlebography is usually available in the venous phase of selective renal arteriography, particularly if large doses of contrast medium are used.

(We routinely perform high dose [30 cc] selective arteriography in all patients with renal carcinoma to evaluate the status of the renal veins which will then be well seen in the venous stage of the study.)

In difficult cases, the knowledge of the type of intrarenal venous involvement may be helpful in differentiating neoplastic from nonneoplastic renal masses such as abscesses. Since renal carcinoma characteristically invades renal veins and other types of masses generally displace or compress these vessels, the renal phlebogram may be of some value in differentiating the lesions. Further experience will be necessary before the importance of this possible finding can be evaluated.

According to Olin and Reuter, the filling of the renal veins may be enhanced during renal phlebography by the use of epinephrine. Ten μg of this drug is introduced through a catheter in the renal artery just prior to performing the renal phlebogram. The subsequent decreased renal blood flow will facilitate retrograde venous flow and give excellent visualization of the renal vein and its intrarenal tributaries.

BIBLIOGRAPHY

Abrams, H. L.: Response of neoplastic renal vessels to epinephrine in man, Radiology 82:217, 1964.

Dos Santos Lamas, A. C., and Pereira-Caldas, J.: Arteriografia da aorta e dos vasos abdominais, Med. contemp. 47:93, 1929.

Evans, J. A.; Monteith, J. C., and Dubilier, W., Jr.: Nephrotomography, Radiology 64, 655, 1955.

Fish, G. W.: Large solitary serous cysts of the kidney, J.A.M.A. 112:514, 1939.

Frimann-Dahl, J.: Normal variations of the left kidney: An anatomic and radiologic study, Acta radiol. 55:207, 1961.

Goldberg, B. B.; Ostrum, B. J., and Isard, H. J.: Nephrosonography: Ultrasound differentiation of renal masses, Radiology 90:1113, 1968.

Greenspan, R. H.; Simon, A. L.; Ricketts, H. J.; Rojas, R. H., and Watson, J. D.: In vivo magnification angiography, Invest. Radiol. 2:419, 1967.

Olin, T. B., and Reuter, S. R.: A pharmacoangiographic method for improving nephrophlebography, Radiology 85:1036, 1965.

Rosenthall, L.: Radionuclide diagnosis of renal cysts and neoplasms using the gamma-ray scintillation camera: Preliminary work, J. Cana. A. Radiol. 17:85, 1966.

Seldinger, S. I.: Catheter replacement of needle in percutaneous arteriography: New technique, Acta radiol. 39:368, 1953.

Shenker, B.: Drip infusion pyelography: Indications and applications in urologic roentgen diagnosis, Radiology 83:12, 1964.

Vestby, G. W.: Percutaneous needle-puncture of renal cysts: New method in therapeutic management, Invest. Radiol. 2:449, 1967.

Von Lichtenberg, A., and Swick, M.: Klinische Prüfung des Uroselectans, Klin. Wchnschr. 8:2089, 1929.

Figure 1.—Normal nephrotomogram.

A, aortic phase of angiogram, anteroposterior projection: This intravenous aortogram demonstrates the abdominal aorta and upper aortic branches. No abnormal vascularity is evident, but visualization of renal vasculature is limited.

B, tomographic cut during nephrogram phase, anteroposterior view: The renal outlines are well demonstrated and normal. The collecting systems are also well seen.

Comment: This nephrotomogram demonstrates the original technique described by Evans *et al.* in which rapid intravenous injection of a large bolus of contrast medium was utilized to obtain the arterial phase. In current practice, drip infusion nephrotomography is used. Arteriography is performed separately in indicated cases (see Figs. 4, 9, 11 and 16).

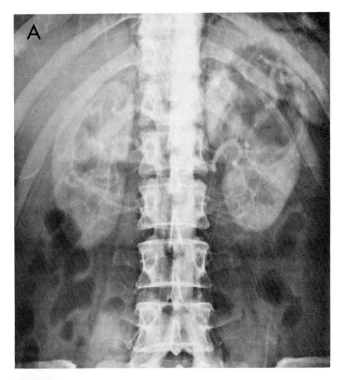

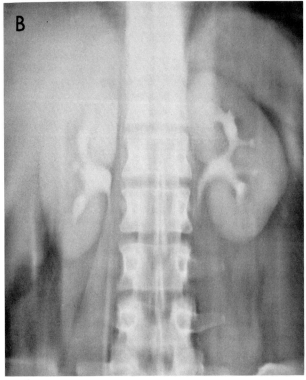

Figure 1 · Normal Nephrotomogram / 13

Figure 2.—Normal nephrotomogram.

Tomographic cut, anteroposterior projection: Demonstrating the renal outlines extremely well. The renal parenchyma is homogeneously opacified. The suprarenal triangular clear spaces are well seen, as are the relationships of the liver and spleen to the kidneys. There is also a so-called splenic hump or dromedary hump of the left kidney (**x**), a normal variant.*

---

* Frimann-Dahl, J.: Normal variations of the left kidney: An anatomic and radiologic study, Acta radiol. 55:207, 1961.

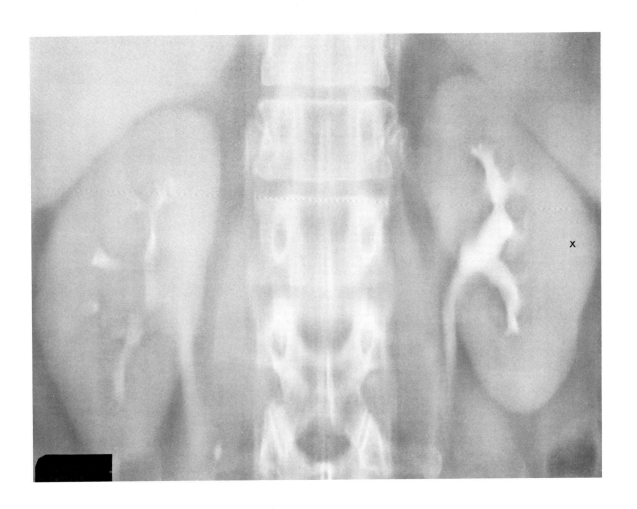

Figure 2 · Normal Nephrotomogram / 15

PART 2

Cystic Disease of the Kidney

Types and Characteristics of Renal Cystic Disease

CYSTIC DISEASE of the kidney, although a relatively common disorder, is a complex, confused subject of conflicting and divergent opinions regarding pathogenesis, classification, morphology and clinical and radiological observations. The relationship of the different varieties of renal cysts to each other is poorly understood. Furthermore it is rather difficult to classify the various forms of cystic disease into clearcut specific categories on the basis of pathogenesis or histologic patterns.

The vast majority of cysts arise in the renal parenchyma and may be single, multiple, unilocular or multilocular. They may be unilateral, bilateral, focal or generalized. A small percentage may originate within the renal sinus (peripelvic); others may be formed from elements of the renal pelvis (pyelogenic).

SIMPLE CYSTS

The term simple cyst is probably preferable to solitary cyst since simple cysts usually do not occur singly even though grossly only one cyst can be observed. Simple cysts may be multiple, unilateral or bilateral. It is said that they occur more often in the lower pole, but in our experience there is no particular site of predilection.

Simple cyst is now generally believed to originate from tubular obstruction and vascular block with ischemia in the obstructed area and subsequent development of a cyst (Hepler). Clinical signs and symptoms are usually few or nonexistent. These cysts are usually discovered as an incidental finding during a medical evaluation. Pain, hematuria and pyuria are rarely significant clinical features.

Urographic appearance depends on the size and location in the renal parenchyma. Centrally located cysts usually produce displacement, compression and distortion on some element of the pelvocalyceal system. Peripherally located cysts may cause contour deformities without affecting the collecting system.

The same urographic appearance may be seen in simple cyst as in neoplasm. Conventional urography therefore is not usually helpful in differentiating cyst from neoplasm.

Occasionally renal cysts exhibit calcification in the form of a thin curved line of calcification along the periphery or margin of the mass (Figs. 13 and 14). Mottled calcification should not be seen in simple cyst but may occur in neoplasm. According to Silverman and Kilhenny and Emmett *et al.,* the occurrence of a neoplasm in the wall of an otherwise simple cyst is a rarity, and we have seen only two such instances in a large series of cases, both correctly diagnosed preoperatively by nephrotomography and angiography (Fig. 60).

PERIPELVIC CYSTS

Peripelvic cysts are situated in the hilus of the kidney intimately associated with the renal pelvis and calyces (Figs. 11 and 12). They may be single or multiple. Unlike the common simple cyst of the kidney, they are not buried within the renal parenchyma. As a result of their hilar location they may compress or displace the renal pelvis and vascular pedicle. If large enough, they may protrude from the renal hilus.

The pathogenesis of these cysts is obscure. It is believed that they originate from the renal sinus rather than from the adjacent renal parenchyma or renal pelvis. A commonly held opinion is that they represent lymphatic cysts which may have developed in areas of lymphatic ectasia secondary to chronic inflammatory changes.

Clinical manifestations are usually lacking. Most of the time these cysts are an incidental finding during examination for an unassociated condition.

On pathologic examination they are bluish thin-walled structures containing yellowish fluid. The cyst walls consist of fibrous tissue with a flattened epithelial cell lining.

Urography usually demonstrates a soft tissue mass in the renal hilus with compression and displacement of the renal pelvis. There may also be some pressure caliectasis. Differentiation of a peripelvic cyst located within the sinus renalis from a centrally located cortical cyst may be difficult. Nephrotomography is sometimes helpful in differentiation. Peripelvic cysts, because they are situated in the renal pelvis or within the renal sinus, are not totally surrounded by opacified renal parenchyma. The margins of such cysts may therefore not be as sharp or distinct as the simple cortical cyst that has a sharp, distinct interface with the opacified parenchyma. The differentiation, however, is more or less academic because the primary issue in such instances is whether the renal mass is benign or malignant. Renal angiography may be necessary to resolve this point.

MULTICYSTIC KIDNEY

This is a distinct pathologic entity and should be distinguished from polycystic kidney, multilocular cystic kidney and multiple simple cysts of the kidney. There is complete replacement of the normal kidney by a conglomeration of cysts of varying sizes that leave no discernible renal parenchyma. The ureter is almost always rudimentary or atretic. The disease is unilateral. There is no familial tendency. Since the kidney cannot be visualized by excretory or retrograde urography, its presence may escape detection until adulthood. Generally, however, multicystic kidney presents as an abdominal mass in an infant (Fig. 18). Congenital hydronephrosis, Wilms' tumor, neuroblastoma and primary retroperitoneal sarcoma are differential diagnostic considerations.

POLYCYSTIC KIDNEY

Polycystic kidney disease is the most important entity to be considered under this category. The pathogenesis of polycystic disease is not known, although over the years a number of hypotheses have been advanced to explain its occurrence. The most commonly accepted theory of the origin of polycystic kidneys is that it represents a failure of the uriniferous tubules (from the embryonic nephrogenic blastema) to connect with the collecting tubules (from the ureteric bud). The disease emerges at two age peaks—infancy and adult life. The infantile and adult forms of the disease, although pathologically similar, are apparently distinct entities. Infantile polycystic kidney disease is invariably fatal, is often associated with other malformations and is inherited as an autosomal recessive. The adult variety is inherited apparently as an autosomal dominant trait but has a variable course. Some patients have a severe form of the disease and present symptoms and signs in early adult life; in others, the disease is discovered accidentally in late adulthood or at autopsy. The great majority of patients present symptoms and signs of the disease in the fourth, fifth and sixth decades. The disease is almost always bilateral (a diagnosis of unilateral polycystic disease is always open to question, although it has been reported to occur). Cysts of the liver are occasionally associated with polycystic kidneys, and rarely cysts of the lungs, pancreas and spleen are observed in these patients. Ten to 20% of patients with polycystic kidney disease have associated intracranial aneurysm, and death from cerebral hemorrhage occurs in about 10% of cases.

The clinical features of the disease may be quite variable including pain, hematuria, renal colic, infection, hypertension and azotemia. The clinical course varies widely depending on the severity of the disease. The effects of hypertension, ruptured intracranial aneurysm or renal insufficiency usually proves fatal.

The classic urographic findings in this disease are large kidneys with lobulated contours. There are striking and frequently bizarre distortions of the pyelocalyceal system, the dominant features of which are stretching, elongation, displacement and splaying of the calyces producing the so-called spiderleg deformity. Occasionally, there is a considerable disparity in the degree of involvement of the two kidneys so that one kidney may appear larger than the other.

In the nephrotomogram, the multiple cysts scattered throughout the renal parenchyma produce a mottled picture with well-defined radiolucent cysts of varying size intermeshed with areas of functioning parenchyma.

Renal arteriography demonstrates stretching and displacement of the interlobar and interlobular arteries by the cysts (Figs. 19 and 20).

Differential diagnostic considerations on conventional urography include fibrolipomatosis, multiple hamartomata (tuberous sclerosis) and bilateral multiple simple cysts.

In a discussion of the radiographic appearance of polycystic disease it should be mentioned that there are instances in which the cysts are relatively small and uniform in size. The urogram therefore may not reflect the classic pattern of pyelocalyceal deformity. In such cases, the true nature of the disease may only be demonstrated by nephrotomography or arteriography.

MEDULLARY SPONGE KIDNEY

This form of cystic disease occurs mainly in adults, although on occasion it is seen in young children and adolescents. The abnormality, which represents cystic dilatation of the distal collecting tubules in the medulla, may be focal, regional or generalized. It may affect only one kidney or both may be involved in varying degree. There are no associated urinary tract abnormalities and there is no familial tendency. Small calculi are prone to form in the dilated ducts of the renal pyramids and pyelonephritis is a not uncommon complication. In many cases the lesion is an unsuspected finding in patients without urinary tract symptoms.

The classic urographic picture shows dilated contrast-filled collecting ducts in the renal pyramids producing a radiating or spraylike pattern. In the more advanced form, well-developed contrast-filled cysts are found in the renal papillae (Fig. 21). At times the differential urographic diagnosis between medullary sponge kidney and the medullary form of papillary necrosis may prove vexing.

MULTILOCULAR CYSTS

This is a rare type of simple cyst of the kidney in which the cystic area is divided by multiple septa separating the cysts into numerous compartments.

Histologically, it is said that multilocular cysts of the kidney develop in a manner comparable to polycystic kidney but that the malformation remains localized to one portion of the organ. The multilocular cyst is sharply set apart from adjacent renal tissue and contains no mature functioning nephrons within its septa.

Multilocular cysts are not associated with abnormalities of other parts of the genitourinary tract, such as atresia of the ureter, as is multicystic kidney.

Urography demonstrates a renal mass which compresses normal renal parenchyma and causes distortion of the pelvis and calyces, as in simple benign cysts. In children, however, multilocular cyst may mimic Wilms' tumor. Nephrotomography may demonstrate the connective tissue septa within the cyst. Cyst puncture and double contrast injection will also show the compartmental character of the cyst (Fig. 22).

ECHINOCOCCUS CYSTS

Hydatid cysts of the kidney occur from infestations by the larval stage of the dog tapeworm. They arise in the cortex and often grow to a large size. Calcification is common either in the wall of the cyst or in the form of daughter cysts (Fig. 23). Sometimes these cysts communicate with a calyx and are then spoken of as open cysts. In such cases retrograde pyelography not only demonstrates the communication but may also disclose the presence of noncalcified daughter cysts. Renal angiography will show displacement of the renal artery branches, as in any other cyst, but late in the capillary phase there may be staining of the wall of the cyst or of daughter cysts. Sometimes a cyst may grow so large as to displace and partially occlude the inferior vena cava.

BIBLIOGRAPHY

Boggs, L. K., and Kimmelstiel, P.: Benign multilocular cystic nephroma: Report of two cases of so-called multilocular cyst of the kidney, J. Urol. 76:530, 1956.

Dalgaard, O. F.: Polycystic Disease of the Kidneys. In Strauss, M. B., and Welt, L. G. (eds.): *Diseases of the Kidney* (Boston: Little, Brown and Co., 1963), p. 907.

Dubilier, W., and Evans, J. A.: Peripelvic cysts of the kidney, Radiology 71:404, 1958.

Emmett, J. L.; Levine, S. R., and Woolner, L. B.: Coexistence of renal cyst and tumor, Brit. J. Urol. 35:403, 1963.

Evans, J. A.: Medullary sponge kidney, Am. J. Roentgenol. 86:119, 1961.

Hepler, A. B.: Solitary cysts of the kidney: A Report of seven cases and observations on the pathogenesis of these cysts, Surg., Gynec. & Obst. 50:668, 1930.

Lindvall, N.: Roentgenologic diagnosis of medullary sponge kidney, Acta radiol. 51: 193, 1959.

Silverman, J. F., and Kilhenny, C.: Tumor in wall of simple renal cyst, Radiology 93: 95, 1969.

Spence, H. M.: Congenital unilateral multicystic kidney: An entity to be distinguished from polycystic kidney disease and other cystic disorders, J. Urol. 74:693, 1955.

Figure 3.—Benign renal cysts; nephrotomograms.

A and **B,** nephrotomograms, anteroposterior views: Demonstrating renal cysts in two patients. Note that each lesion is homogeneously lucent, sharply marginated and has a thin wall (**a**). Also present is a sharp spur at the interface with the kidney (**b**).

Comment: The nephrotomograms in these two cases clearly demonstrate the radiographic criteria of a benign cyst. It must be emphasized that *all* of the criteria of a cyst must be present if this diagnosis is to be made, particularly the *thin wall*. In our experience an image with a wall as depicted in these cases has not been shown to represent a lesion other than a benign cyst. Cortical spurs (**b**) are helpful though not infallible evidence of benignity.*

---

* Olsson, O.: Renal Tumor and Cyst. In Abrams, H. L. (ed.): *Angiography* (Boston: Little, Brown and Company, 1961), Vol. II, p. 557.

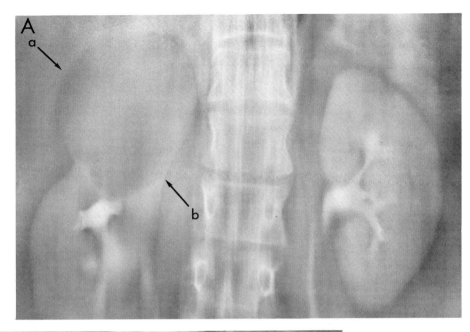

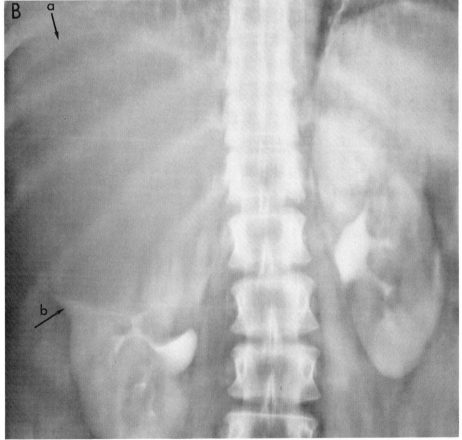

Figure 3 · Benign Cysts: Nephrotomograms / 25

Figure 4.—Intrarenal cyst.

A, nephrotomogram, anteroposterior view: Delineating a lucent well-defined lesion in the lower pole of the left kidney (**arrows**). The lower pole calyx is displaced posteriorly and not visualized on this "tomographic cut." A few small calcifications are seen in the spleen.

B, selective left renal arteriogram, arterial phase, anteroposterior projection: Revealing stretching of the intrarenal vessels over the mass in the lower pole of the kidney. No abnormal appearing vessels can be seen.

C, same study, nephrogram phase: Demonstrating a well marginated lucent defect in the lower pole of the kidney.

A 58-year-old man entered the hospital for lower urinary tract symptoms. The mass in the left kidney was considered to be a simple benign intrarenal cyst and it was not further investigated. One year later, the patient had a followup urogram which showed no change in the appearance of the cyst.

Comment: The lesion in this case is wholly intrarenal. Thus demonstration of a thin wall is not possible. A definite diagnosis of a simple benign cyst cannot therefore be made by nephrotomography alone, and in such a case, confirmatory angiography should be obtained in this type of deep-seated lesion. The angiogram demonstrates the avascular nature of the lesion with no evidence of tumor vascularity and confirms its benignity.

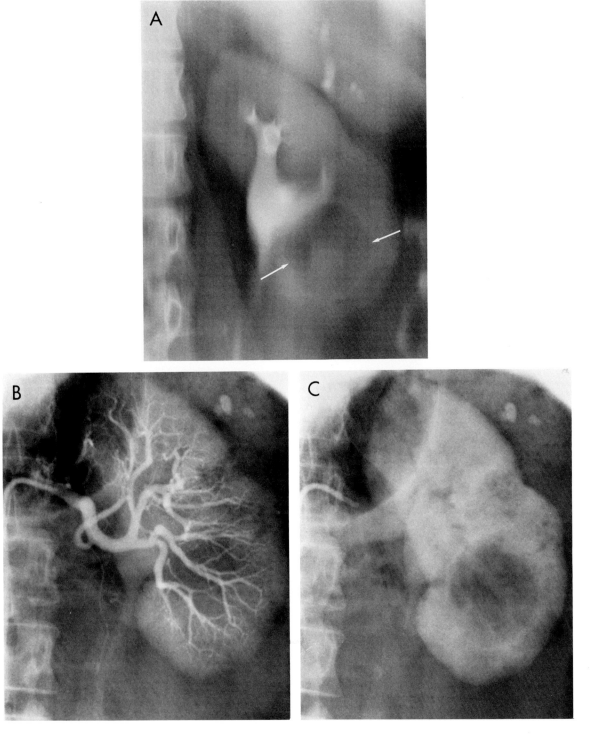

Figure 4 · Intrarenal Cyst / 27

Figure 5.—Benign renal cyst.

A, intravenous urogram, anteroposterior view: Showing a large mass occupying the upper pole of the right kidney (**arrows**) that causes flattening and splaying of the upper pole calyx (**x**).

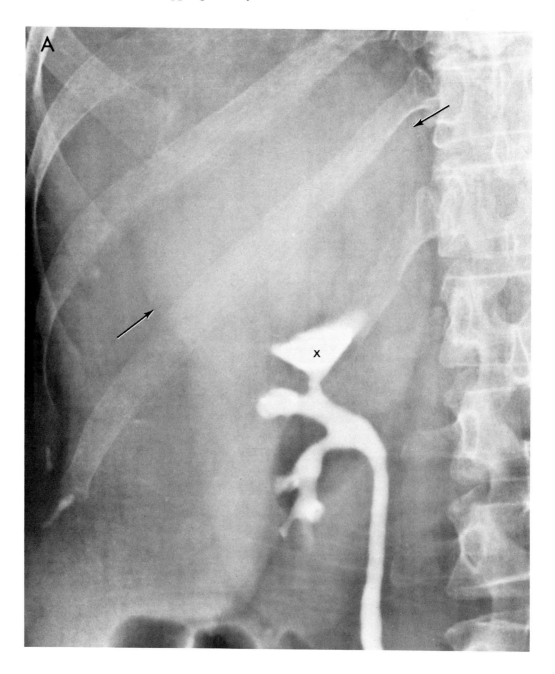

B, nephrotomogram anteroposterior view: Delineating a 10 cm diameter mass at the upper pole of the right kidney which demonstrates all criteria necessary for a diagnosis of benign cyst. The mass is well margined, homogeneously lucent, has a thin wall (**a**) and sharp interface with the kidney (**b**).

The patient, a 57-year-old woman, consulted her physician because of urgency and dysuria. The renal cyst was an incidental finding during the investigation of the patient's lower urinary tract complaints.

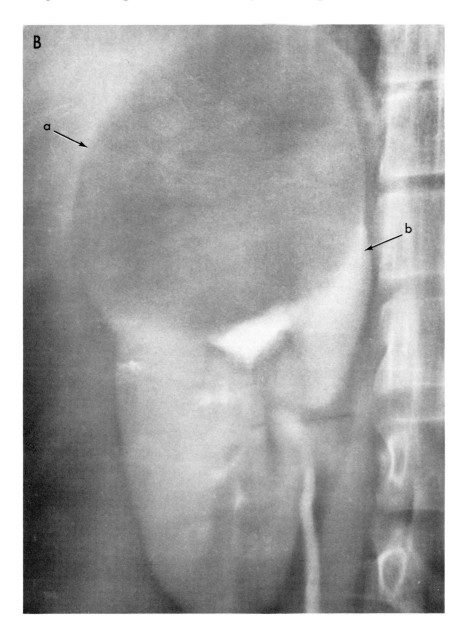

Figure 5 · Benign Cyst / 29

Figure 6.—Bilateral simple benign renal cysts.

A, intravenous urogram, anteroposterior view: Disclosing a large mass at the upper pole of each kidney, with calyceal distortions of upper pole calyces bilaterally. Multiple gallstones are superimposed on the upper half of the right kidney.

B, nephrotomogram, tomographic cut: Revealing that both lesions are simple benign cysts (**arrows**). The lesions are well marginated, homogeneously lucent, thin-walled and have a sharp interface with each kidney.

A 54-year-old woman entered the hospital with a history of episodes of urinary frequency and mild dysuria. Surgery was not thought to be indicated for the bilateral renal cysts, so the patient was discharged from the hospital. Six years later, she had a transitional cell carcinoma of the left renal pelvis which required a left ureteronephrectomy. A simple benign cyst occupying the upper pole of the left kidney was an incidental finding, confirming the accuracy of the roentgen examination interpreted six years previously.

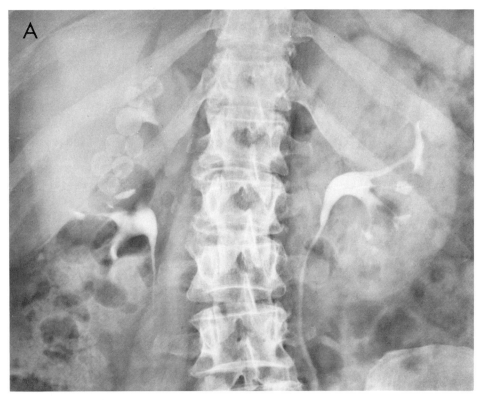

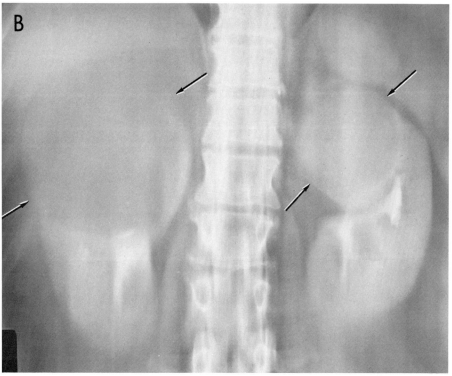

Figure 6 · Bilateral Benign Cysts / 31

Figure 7.—Benign simple cyst of the kidney.

A, selective left renal arteriogram, arterial phase, anteroposterior projection: Revealing a completely avascular mass in the upper pole of the kidney with characteristic compression and displacement of intrarenal vessels.

B, same study, nephrogram phase: Demonstrating the uniformly lucent mass with thin wall, sharp interface with the kidney and well-defined cortical spur (**arrow**),* all findings typical of benign cyst.

This 56-year-old woman entered the hospital because of left flank pain. At surgery a large cyst of the upper pole of the left kidney was discovered and unroofed.

---

* Dautrebande, J.; Duckett, C., and Roy, P.: Claw sign of cortical cysts in renal arteriography, J. Canad. A. Radiol. 18:240, 1967.

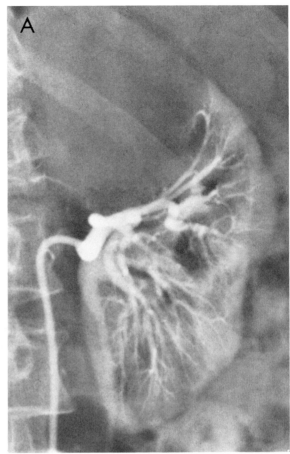

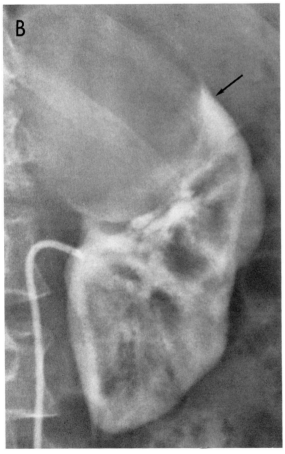

Figure 7 · Benign Cyst: Arteriograms / 33

Figure 8.—Simple cyst of the renal cortex, well demonstrated in oblique projection.

A, selective left renal arteriogram, anteroposterior projection: Clearly demonstrating the vessels to the kidney. Note branches from the main renal artery, including the inferior adrenal artery (**a**) and a capsular artery (**b**). Intrarenal arteries in the lateral margin of the midportion of the kidney show some slight stretching and distortion. Note the defect in the nephrogram at the lateral margin of the kidney (**c**). However, the renal mass is not well defined.

B, same study, left posterior oblique projection: In which the size and extent of the left renal mass can be fully appreciated (**d**). It is completely avascular and exhibits a sharp, well-defined interface with the normal renal parenchyma. A typical spur, frequently associated with a simple cyst, is seen at the inferior margin (**arrow**).

The patient, a man of 76, was hospitalized because of prostatism.

Comment: This case demonstrates well the importance of the oblique view in the study of renal masses. The extent of the renal mass and its benign characteristics were not fully appreciated in the anteroposterior projection, whereas the oblique projection clearly established the size and character of the lesion.

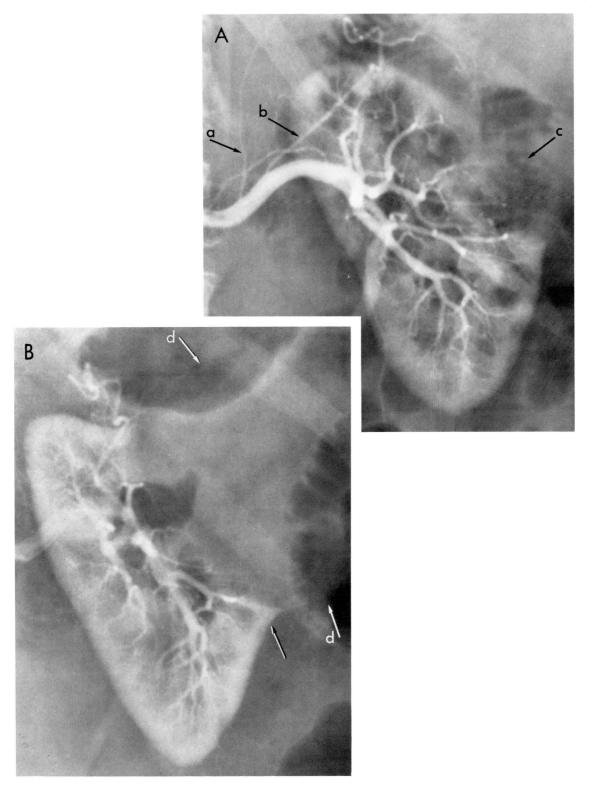

Figure 8 · Simple Cyst of Cortex: Arteriograms / 35

Figure 9.—Large benign cyst; nephrotomography and arteriography.

A, intravenous urogram, anteroposterior view: Showing a large mass occupying the lower pole of the left kidney and causing pressure and upward displacement of the lower pole calyces and renal pelvis.

B, nephrotomogram, tomographic cut: Demonstrating characteristic findings of a large renal cyst with thin walls, well-defined borders, sharp interface with normal parenchyma and cortical spurs (**arrows**).

C, selective left renal arteriogram, anteroposterior view: Showing the mass to be totally avascular.

A woman of 72 was hospitalized with a history of vague abdominal cramps and loose stools.

Comment: The combined approach of selective arteriography and nephrotomography increases overall radiographic diagnostic accuracy in the study of renal masses.

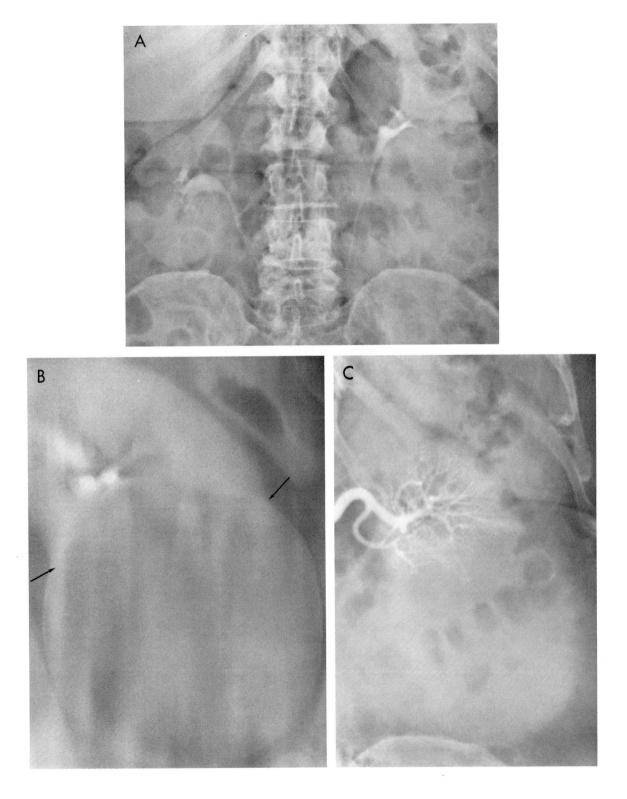

Figure 9 · Large Benign Cyst: Combined Study / 37

Figure 10.—Simple benign cyst: cyst puncture.

A, intravenous urogram, anteroposterior exposure: Showing a large mass (**arrows**) occupying the lower pole of the left kidney. A duplicated collecting system is present.

B, selective left renal arteriogram, anteroposterior view: Indicating that the intrarenal vasculature is normal, while the large mass extending from the lower pole is entirely avascular. The angiographic appearance is typical of renal cyst. The true lower pole of the kidney can be seen through the overlying cyst (**arrows**).

(*Continued* on p. 40.)

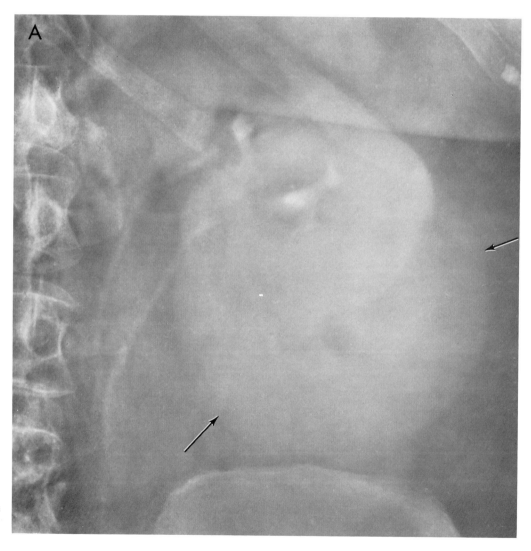

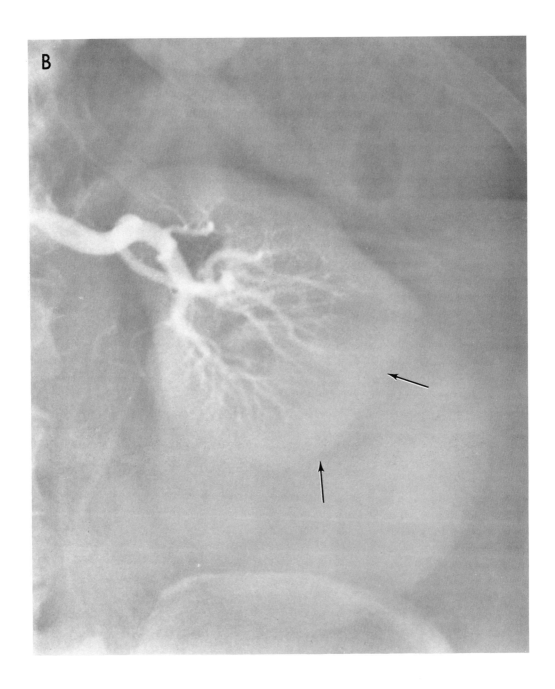

Figure 10 · Simple Benign Cyst: Cyst Puncture / 39

Figure 10 (cont.).—Simple benign cyst: cyst puncture.

C, film after percutaneous cyst puncture and instillation of contrast medium, anteroposterior projection: Showing the cyst with smooth walls and no evidence of filling defects. The metallic density in the middle of the cyst is the needle seen on end.

D, triple contrast study; film taken with patient upright after instillation of 5 cc of Pantopaque (**a**), 20 cc of Renografin (**b**) and 10 cc of air (**c**). No filling defects or significant irregularities of the wall are demonstrated. The cyst is partially collapsed since 300 cc of clear fluid has been removed.

A 53-year-old man entered the hospital because of low back pain.

Comment: The 300 cc of fluid that was removed was clear and contained no malignant cells. Multiple films were obtained in various projections so that all contours of the cyst might be visualized. The Pantopaque was instilled in the hope that it would lead to permanent collapse of the cyst and thereby the procedure would be therapeutic as well as contributing to diagnosis.

Figure 10, courtesy of Dr. Plinio Rossi, St. Vincent's Hospital, New York.

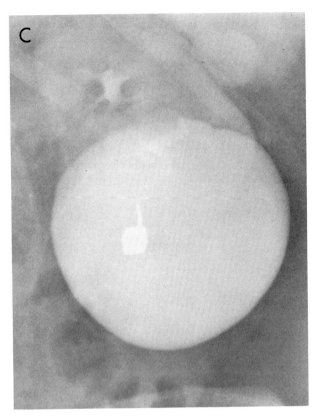

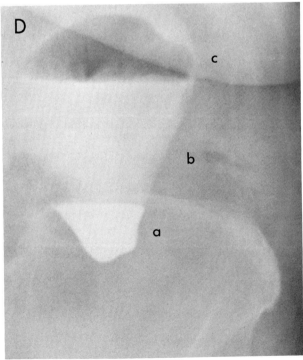

Figure 10 · Simple Benign Cyst: Cyst Puncture / 41

Figure 11.—Peripelvic cyst.

A, intravenous urogram, anteroposterior view of right kidney: Revealing a peripelvic mass inferior to the renal pelvis, causing pressure on the pelvis and middle pole infundibular structures (**arrows**), and displacing the lower pole calyx which is only partly filled laterally (**crossed arrow**).

B, selective right renal arteriogram, arterial phase, right posterior oblique projection: Revealing that the large peripelvic mass is essentially avascular. A number of renal artery branches to the cortex of the kidney at the lower pole are draped about the mass (**arrows**). No abnormal appearing vessels, however, are visualized.

C, same study, nephrogram phase: Demonstrating that lesion is totally avascular and lucent and bulging out from the hilus of the kidney (**arrow**). Lesion is characteristic of large, avascular benign peripelvic cyst.

The patient, a man of 68, was hospitalized with symptoms of prostatism. He underwent prostatectomy. His right kidney was not explored because of the lesion's characteristic appearance of a benign cyst.

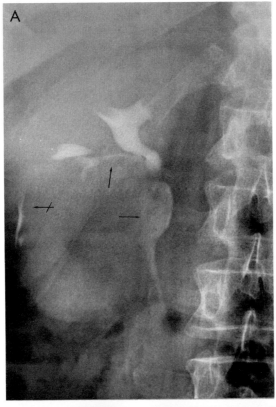

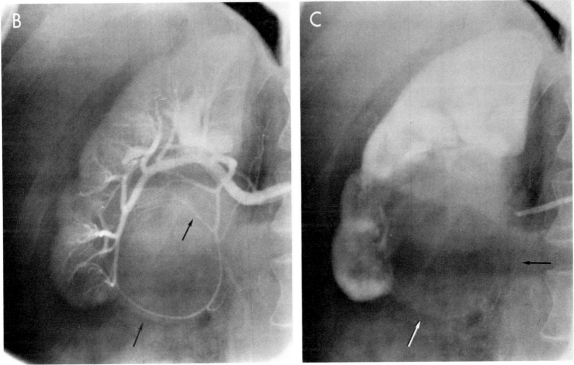

Figure 11 · Peripelvic Cyst / 43

Figure 12.—Peripelvic cyst and fibromuscular dysplasia of the renal artery.

A, intravenous urogram, anteroposterior view: Showing that the axis of the upper pole of the right kidney, including the superior calyceal group, has been shifted laterally. The renal margin medially above the renal pelvis is indistinct, suggesting the possibility of a mass medial to the kidney. The mass can barely be seen in this study.

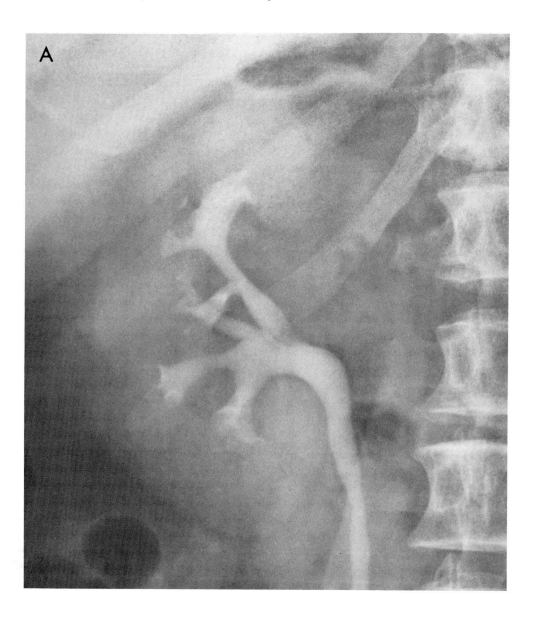

B, nephrotomogram: Clearly demonstrating a mass medial to the kidney just above the renal pelvis (**arrows**). The margins are smooth and the wall is thin, but further characteristics are not well defined. The lesion appears to be rather "dense" because it is surrounded by lucent perirenal and peripelvic fat and because of photographic enhancement.

(*Continued* on p. 46.)

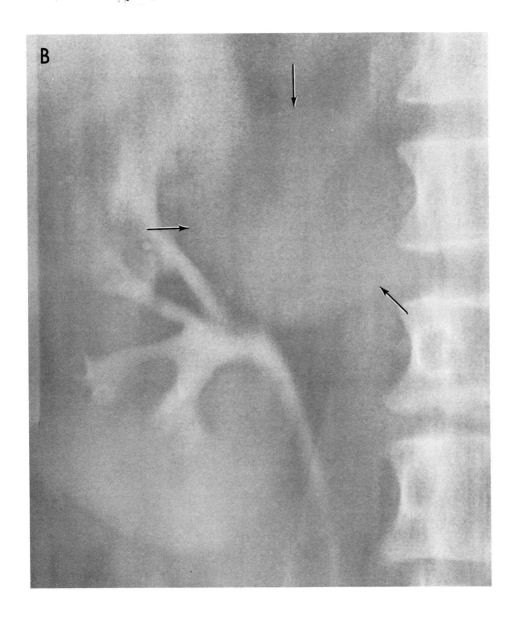

Figure 12 · Peripelvic Cyst with Fibromuscular Dysplasia / 45

Figure 12 (cont.).—Peripelvic cyst and fibromuscular dysplasia of the renal artery.

C, selective right renal arteriogram: Revealing branches of the main renal artery stretched over a peripelvic mass (**arrow**). The mass is avascular and has the typical appearance of a peripelvic cyst. Changes of fibromuscular dysplasia involve the renal artery and its branches (**a**). The inferior adrenal artery is displaced medially by the cyst (**b**).

A 57-year-old woman was hospitalized for study prior to gynecologic surgery. She did not have hypertension.

Comment: The combination of nephrotomography and renal arteriography established the diagnosis, and it was decided that renal surgery was not indicated. The presence of fibromuscular dysplasia without hypertension is of interest but not rare; we have seen it on a number of occasions.

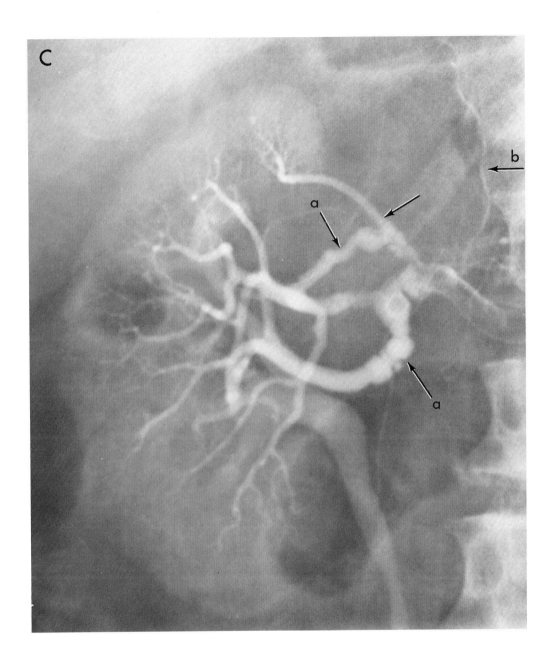

Figure 12 · Peripelvic Cyst with Fibromuscular Dysplasia / 47

Figure 13.—Calcified cyst of the kidney.

Intravenous urogram, anteroposterior projection: Delineating a mass with curvilinear calcification in its wall, seen at the upper pole of the left kidney.

A man of 59 for four years had been known to have a calcified mass in the upper abdomen, thought to be a pancreatic cyst. On surgical exploration a calcified renal cyst was found.

Comment: The presence of calcium in the wall of a renal mass does not help in deciding whether it is benign or malignant. This type of calcification is found in benign simple cysts as well as malignant lesions. A lesion with such calcification must be considered malignant until proven otherwise.* Of course, calcification in the center of a renal mass rules out a simple cyst and makes neoplasm very likely.

---

* Arkless, R.: Cyst-like calcification in renal cell carcinomas, Clin. Radiol. 17:397, 1966.

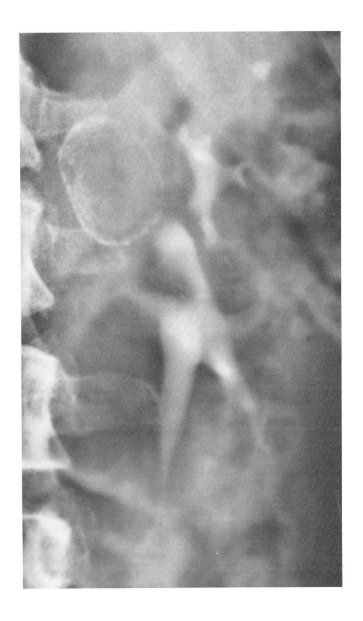

Figure 13 · Calcified Renal Cyst / 49

Figure 14.—Calcified cyst of the kidney.

 A, left retrograde pyelogram, anteroposterior view: Showing a large mass at the lower pole of the slightly rotated left kidney. The mass has a thin calcific wall (**arrows**).

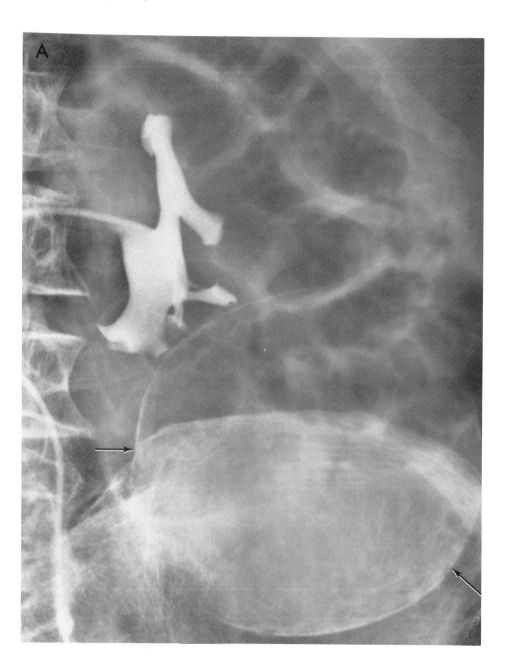

B, nephrotomogram, anteroposterior projection: Clearly demonstrating the mass and calcific wall. The lesion has the appearance of a benign cyst but because of calcium in the wall, this diagnosis cannot be made with certainty on the basis of this study alone (see Comment, Fig. 13). The cyst was punctured, aspirated and then filled with opaque medium. The roentgenograms revealed a lesion with the smooth-walled characteristic of cysts. The aspirated fluid was clear amber and cytologically negative.

The patient, a man of 78, entered the hospital because of symptoms of prostatism.

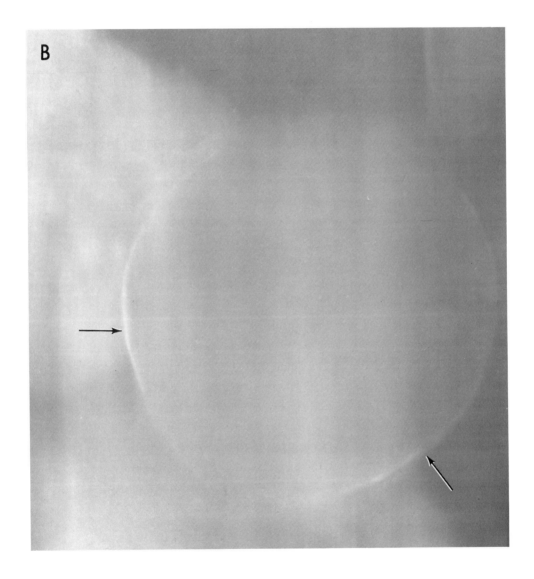

Figure 14 · Calcified Renal Cyst / 51

Figure 15.—Benign cyst in a malrotated kidney.

A, nephrotomogram, tomographic cut, anteroposterior view: Revealing a radiolucent mass of 5 cm diameter (**arrows**) occupying the center of a malrotated kidney. The lesion has smooth contours, is radiolucent and is entirely intrarenal.

B, selective right renal arteriogram, anteroposterior projection: The main renal artery originated from the aorta at the level of the third lumbar vertebra. The intrarenal vessels are somewhat distorted because of malrotation. The major branches are stretched and draped around the mass, which is totally avascular. The renal pelvis is rotated laterally (**arrow**). (The most medial portion of the cortex was supplied by a small branch from the aorta.)

A 58-year-old woman was hospitalized because of a right lower quadrant mass. An intravenous urogram revealed a low-positioned, malrotated kidney which appeared to contain a mass, and the radiographic studies shown here were carried out. Because the radiographic diagnosis was benign cyst, surgery was not performed. The right lower quadrant mass was considered to be an anomalous low-lying kidney.

Comment: The combination of nephrotomography and selective arteriography established that this lesion was benign. Also, because the renal artery originated from the aorta at the level of the third lumbar vertebra, it became clear that the cyst was not responsible for the abnormal rotation and position of the kidney but that a congenital malrotation was present.

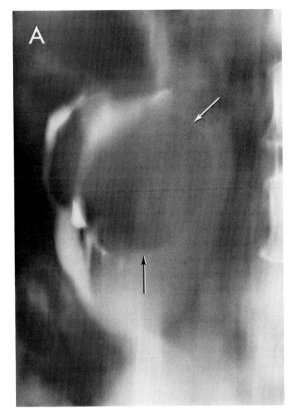

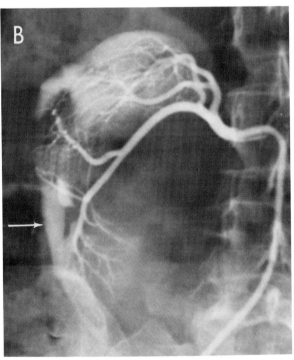

Figure 15 · Benign Cyst in Malrotated Kidney / 53

Figure 16.—Multiple cysts of the kidney.

A, intravenous urogram, anteroposterior projection: Demonstrating distortion of the collecting system by a number of large masses (x) in the right kidney.

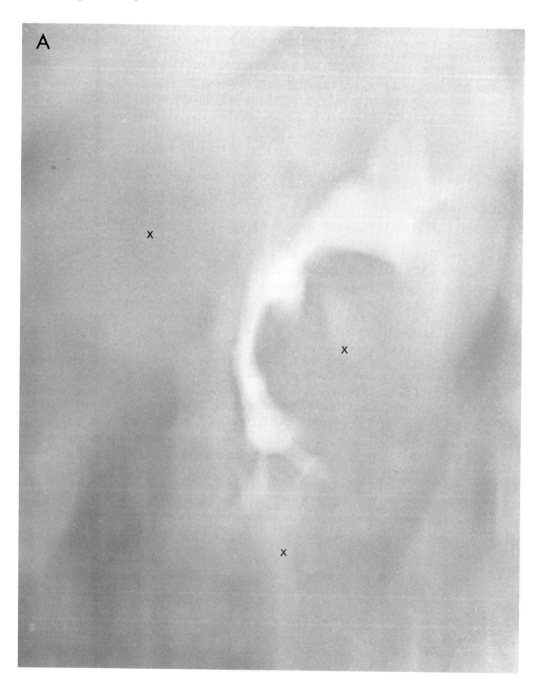

B, nephrotomogram, tomographic cut: Revealing three large masses (**arrows**) having the radiographic appearance of benign cortical cysts. Other cysts were seen at other tomographic levels. (The cysts appear to be a little more dense than usual due to photographic enhancement.)

(*Continued* on p. 56.)

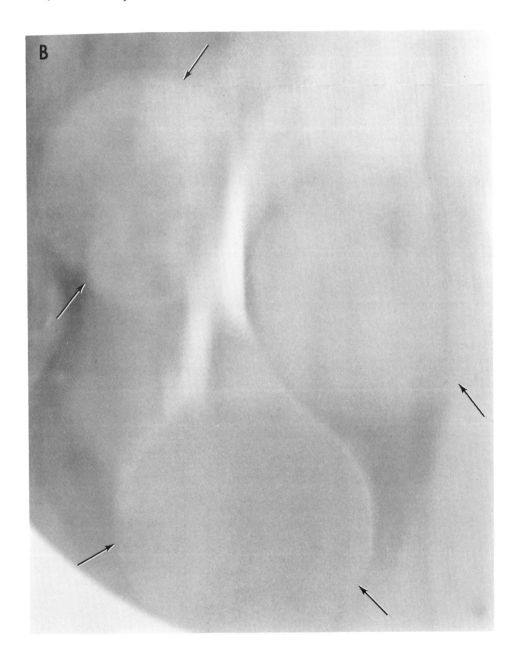

Figure 16 · Multiple Cysts / 55

Figure 16 (cont.).—Multiple cysts of the kidney.

C, selective right renal arteriogram, late arterial phase, anteroposterior exposure: Showing intrarenal vessels displaced and draped around the several renal cysts (**x**). The only sizable areas of functioning renal tissue lie at the upper pole medially and the lower pole laterally (**y**).

The patient, a man of 73, was hospitalized because of symptoms of prostatism.

Comment: A combination of nephrotomography and arteriography is required in cases of multiple masses of the kidney to make certain that all are benign. Because of the distortion caused by these masses and their multiplicity, the combined method is usually necessary to rule out an associated malignant lesion.

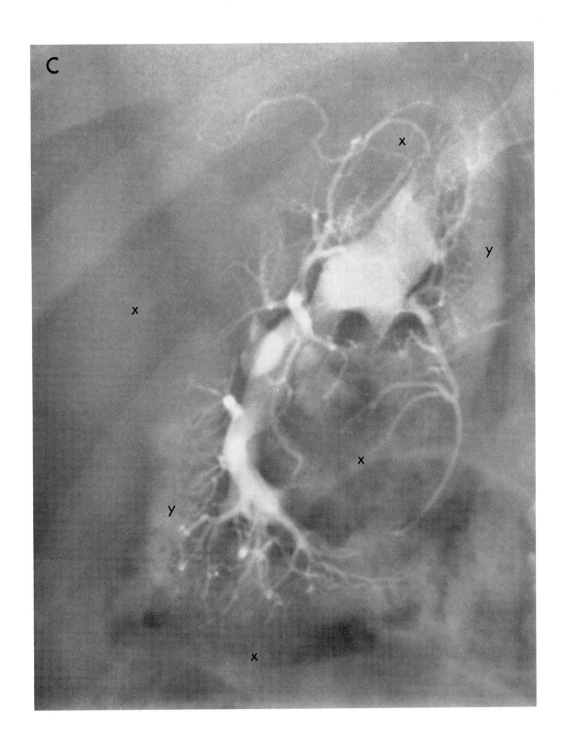

Figure 16 · Multiple Cysts / 57

Figure 17.—Multiple cysts in both kidneys.

A, intravenous urogram, anteroposterior projection: Showing bilateral calyceal distortions and contour irregularities that suggest multiple masses in both kidneys.

B, aortogram, arterial phase, anteroposterior exposure: With midstream aortic injection demonstrating displacement of vessels in both kidneys around multiple avascular masses. Mild diffuse atherosclerosis of the aorta and renal vessels is evident.

(*Continued* on p. 60.)

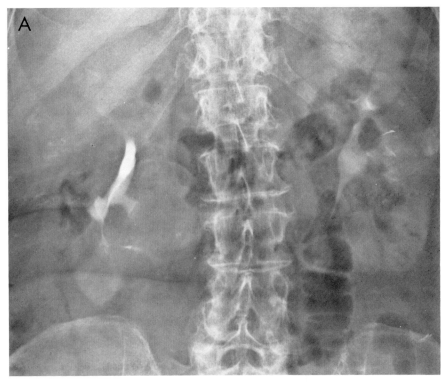

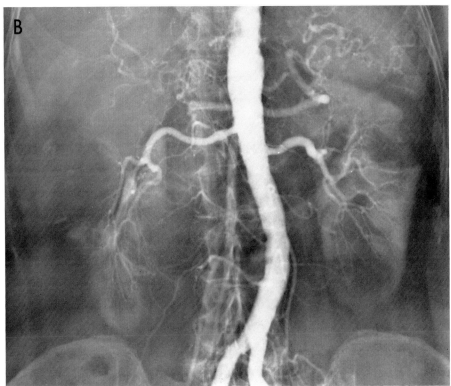

Figure 17 · Bilateral Multiple Cysts / 59

Figure 17 (cont.).—Multiple cysts of both kidneys.

    C, aortogram (same study as **B**), early nephrogram phase: Demonstrating multiple large cysts in both kidneys that cause a significant decrease in amount of functioning parenchyma.

(*Continued* on p. 62.)

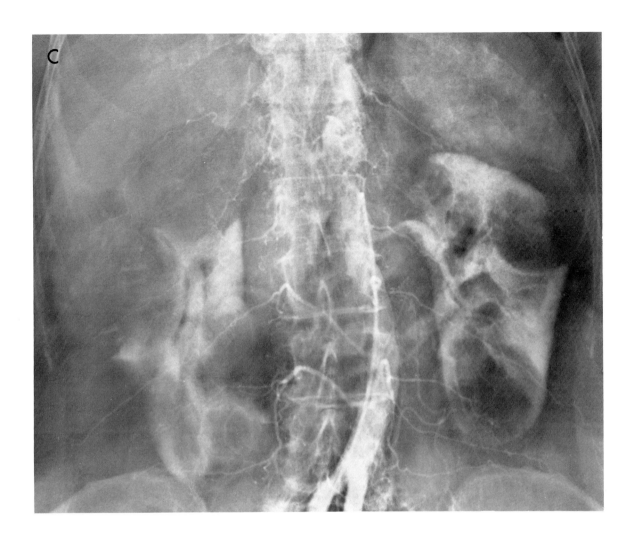

C

Figure 17 · Bilateral Multiple Cysts / 61

Figure 17 (cont.).—Multiple cysts of both kidneys.

D, nephrotomogram, tomographic cut, right kidney, oblique view: Showing at least three large cysts (**arrows**) at the level of this tomographic cut. Each is well marginated and lucent and exhibits a very thin wall, diagnostic of benign cysts. At other tomographic levels more cysts were demonstrated.

E, nephrotomogram, left kidney: Indicating at least three large cysts (**arrows**). Additional cysts in this kidney were seen at other levels.

A man of 66 had symptoms of prostatism. There was no history of hypertension.

Comment: Multiple cysts of the kidneys usually have no clinical significance, although occasionally they cause mild flank pain. It is important, however, to rule out associated renal malignancy.

Differentiation of multiple benign cysts from polycystic kidneys is usually readily made on the basis of clinical history and urography but occasionally is extremely difficult. Polycystic kidneys usually are familial, associated with hypertension or renal insufficiency, and show gross enlargement of the kidneys and wider longitudinal spread of the calyces. Also, the cysts are very variable in size, and there is no totally uninvolved parenchyma, as is present in this case.

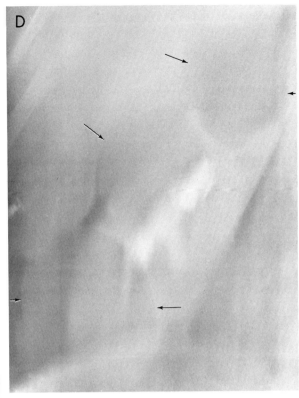

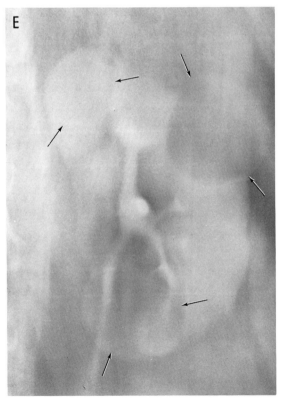

Figure 17 · Bilateral Multiple Cysts / 63

Figure 18.—Multicystic kidney.

A, intravenous urogram, anteroposterior projection: Revealing a mass in the right side of the abdomen with displacement of bowel gas toward the midline. The right kidney is not demonstrated.

B, surgical specimen: A large mass made up entirely of a conglomeration of cysts of varying sizes. There is no normal renal tissue and the renal pelvis cannot be identified. The ureter was atretic.

The patient was a newborn infant with a large right flank mass.

Comment: Multicystic kidney occurs unilaterally. It generally presents as an abdominal mass in an infant but may not be discovered until adulthood.* The total absence of function demonstrated on the excretory urogram differentiates it from most cases of Wilms' tumor and neuroblastoma. Its differentiation from congenital hydronephrosis might, however, be difficult on urography when the hydronephrotic kidney lacks a rim of functioning parenchyma (crescent sign) or is not visualized on delayed films.

Figure 18, courtesy of Grossman, H.; Winchester, P. H., and Chisari, F. V.: Roentgenographic classification of renal cystic disease, Am. J. Roentgenol. 104:319, 1968.

* Bartley, O.; Cederbom, G., and Hegnell, B.: Multicystic renal disease in an adult, Acta radiol. (diag.) 6:424, 1967.
Lalli, A. F.: Multicystic kidney disease, Radiology 89:857, 1967.

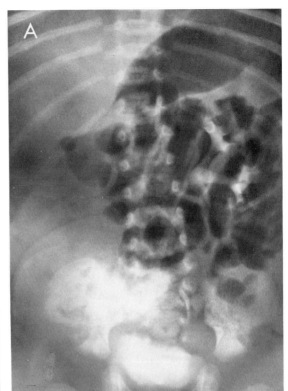

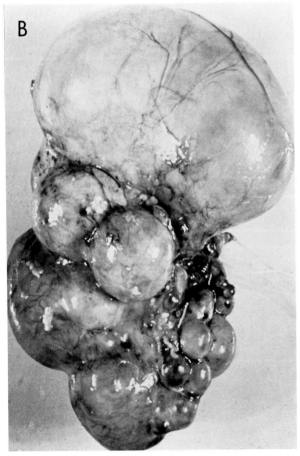

Figure 18 · Multicystic Kidney / 65

Figure 19.—Polycystic kidneys.

A, bilateral retrograde pyelogram, anteroposterior exposure: Showing huge kidneys, with the calyces stretched and distorted by multiple large masses. Each kidney measures 20 cm in its longitudinal axis.

(*Continued* on p. 68.)

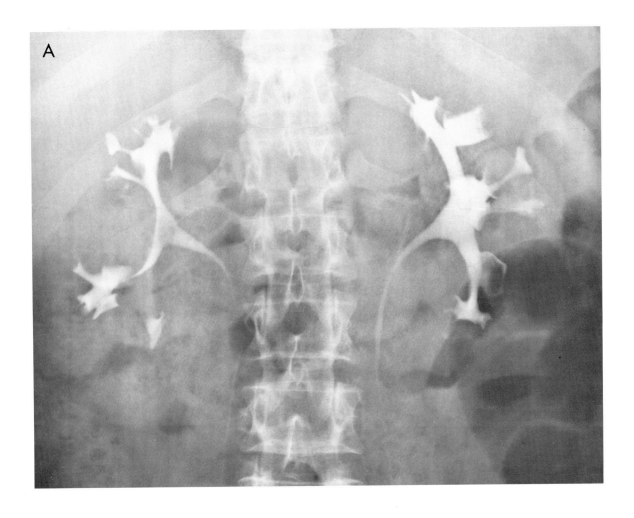

Figure 19 · Polycystic Kidneys / 67

Figure 19 (cont.).—Polycystic kidneys.

B, right selective renal angiogram, arterial phase, anteroposterior exposure: Demonstrating displacement of intrarenal branches by multiple large and small masses and decrease of terminal branching. No abnormal vascularity is seen.

C, same study, nephrogram phase: Showing the parenchyma to be riddled with large, medium-sized and small radiolucencies indicating cysts of the kidney. The nephrogram nicely demonstrates the classic Swiss-cheese findings in polycystic kidneys.

A 30-year-old man was studied because of right flank pain. His mother had polycystic kidneys.

Comment: This case demonstrates the classic findings and history of polycystic disease. The angiograms help to establish the diagnosis and the stage and severity of the disease.*

---

* Ettinger, A.; Kahn, P. C., and Wise, H. M.: The importance of selective renal angiography in the diagnosis of polycystic disease, J. Urol. 102:156, 1969; Cornell, S. H.: Angiography in polycystic disease of the kidneys, J. Urol. 103:24, 1970.

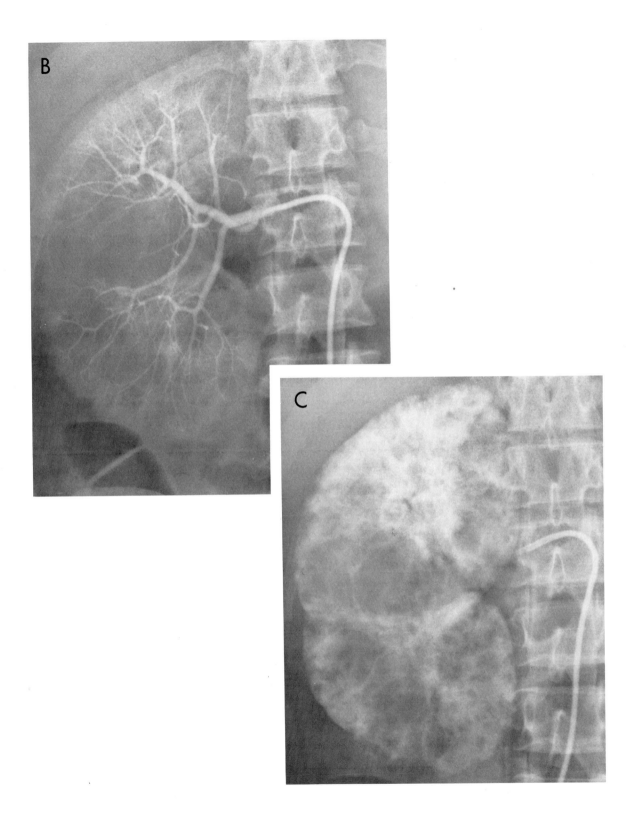

Figure 19 · Polycystic Kidneys / 69

Figure 20.—Polycystic kidneys.

A, right retrograde pyelogram, anteroposterior exposure: Revealing enlargement of the kidney with spread and distortion of the collecting system. The outline of the kidney is not well seen; it measures 19.5 cm in length. There were similar findings in the left kidney.

B, selective right renal arteriogram, arterial phase, anteroposterior projection: Delineating main renal arteries of normal appearance, but showing stretching and displacement of the intrarenal branches and decrease of terminal branching.

(*Continued* on p. 72.)

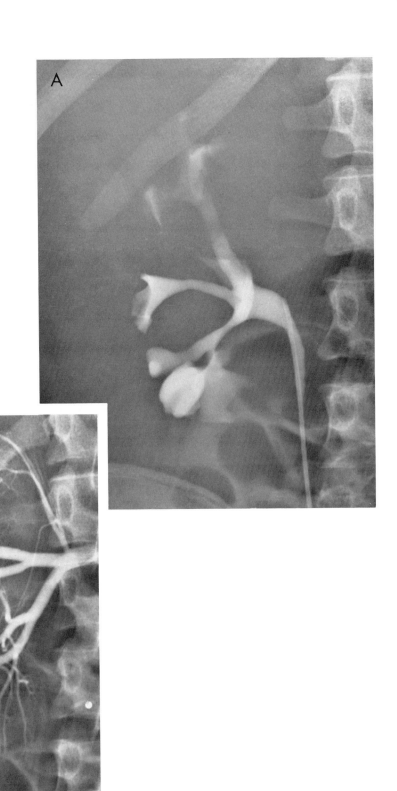

Figure 20 · Polycystic Kidneys / 71

Figure 20 (cont.).—Polycystic kidneys.

C, same study, nephrogram phase: Showing spongy irregular nephrogram. Most of the cysts are small to tiny in size, with no really large cysts evident. All portions of the nephrogram are involved.

A youth of 19 was hospitalized because of trauma to the right flank. An intravenous urogram revealed enlarged kidneys and evidence of multiple masses.

Comment: This is an example of an early stage of polycystic kidney disease. The patient did not have hypertension or laboratory evidence of renal disease, and the diagnosis was incidental to study for possible renal injury. The nephrogram phase of the angiogram (**C**) beautifully demonstrates the numerous small cysts in this patient's kidney.

Figure 20, courtesy of Dr. E. J. Ferris, Boston University Medical Center, Boston.

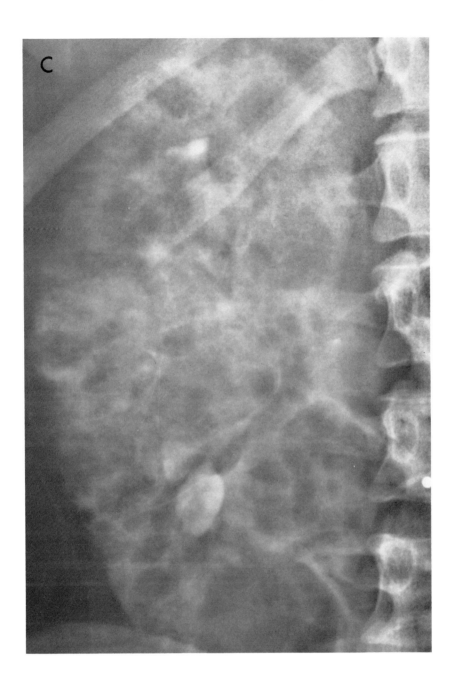

C

Figure 20 · Polycystic Kidneys / 73

Figure 21.—Adult medullary sponge kidney.

A, intravenous urogram, anteroposterior view: Revealing striking collections and concentrations of contrast medium in the renal medullary substances of both kidneys. The left kidney is considerably larger than the right, probably merely an expression of the hemihypertrophy of the left side of the body (see clinical history). The collections of contrast medium outside the collecting systems appear to be in dilated tubules and cystlike structures in the renal papillae and pyramids.

B, nephrotomogram, right kidney, anteroposterior projection: Demonstrating in graphic manner the varying sizes of contrast-filled medullary cysts and dilated tubules. Many minor calyces are large and deeply cupped, reflecting the large size of the renal papillae.

C, nephrotomogram, left kidney: Showing similar but more pronounced findings. The large cystic areas are well demonstrated.

A man of 29 consulted his physician because of occasional occipital headaches and a sense of tension. His health was otherwise good. Physical examination revealed mild left body hemihypertrophy and no other abnormality.

Comment: This is the most pronounced example of medullary sponge kidney in our experience. When first seen the patient had no urinary tract symptoms. Over the next ten years, however, he had mild episodes of pyelonephritis. It is interesting that on a urographic study ten years after the initial examination there was no change in the appearance of either kidney.

Figure 21, courtesy of Evans, J. A.: Medullary sponge kidney, Am. J. Roentgenol. 86:119, 1961.

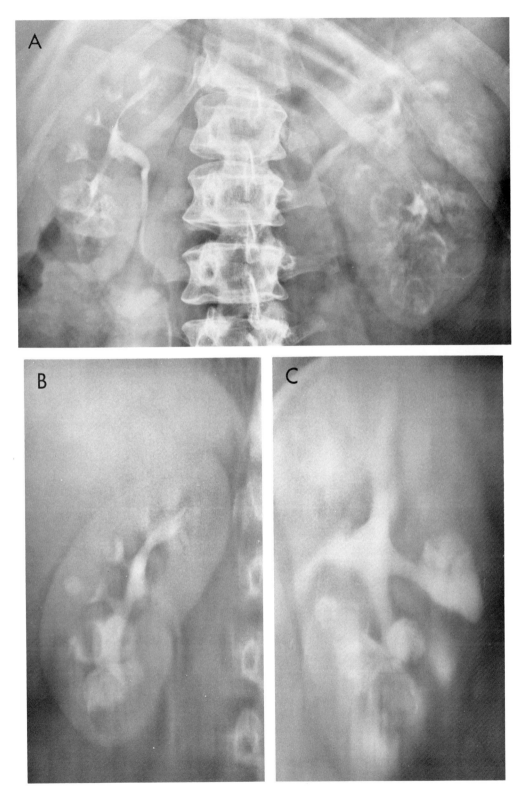

Figure 21 · Medullary Sponge Kidney / 75

Figure 22.—Multilocular cyst.

A, intravenous urogram, anteroposterior exposure: Delineating a large mass (**arrows**) occupying the upper pole of the left kidney and displacing the kidney inferiorly and medially.

B, abdominal film following cyst puncture, aspiration and injection of air and an opaque contrast medium, anteroposterior view: Showing a large cyst which is multiseptated, as can be seen from the numerous loculated gas collections (**arrows**).

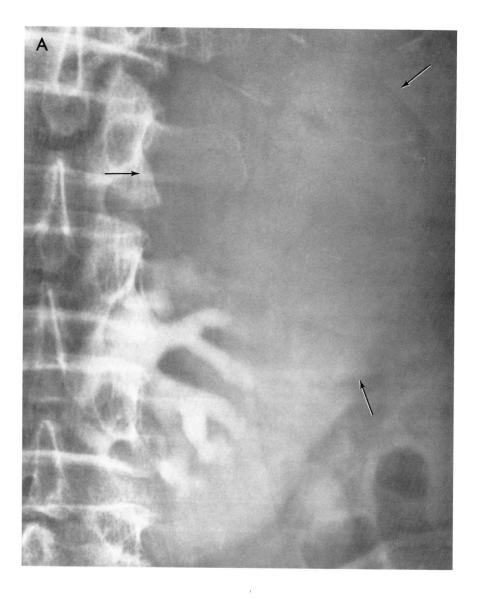

The patient, a man of 61 years, was first seen because of hematuria caused by a left ureteral calculus which passed spontaneously. Examination disclosed a large left abdominal mass. Excretory urography revealed a large upper pole mass, and nephrotomography showed the mass to be a cyst. Because of his poor cardiac status, surgery was not done. The cyst was aspirated and clear fluid obtained; cytologic examination of the fluid revealed no malignant cells. Instillation of opaque contrast agent and some gas allowed clear radiographic demonstration of the multilocular nature of the cyst.

Figure 22, courtesy of Dr. J. A. Becker, State University of New York, Downstate Medical Center, New York.

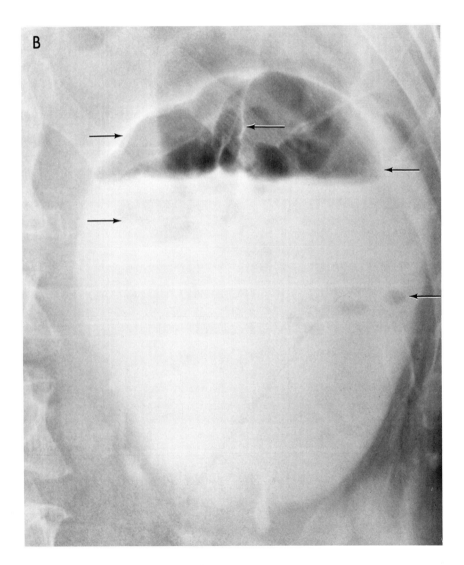

Figure 22 · Multilocular Cyst / 77

Figure 23.—Echinococcus cyst.

    A, intravenous urogram, anteroposterior projection: Revealing a normal left kidney and a large mass involving most of the right kidney. Only a portion of the superior pole calyx can be seen (**upper arrow**). Curvilinear calcification is present along the periphery of the inferior margin of the mass (**lower arrows**).

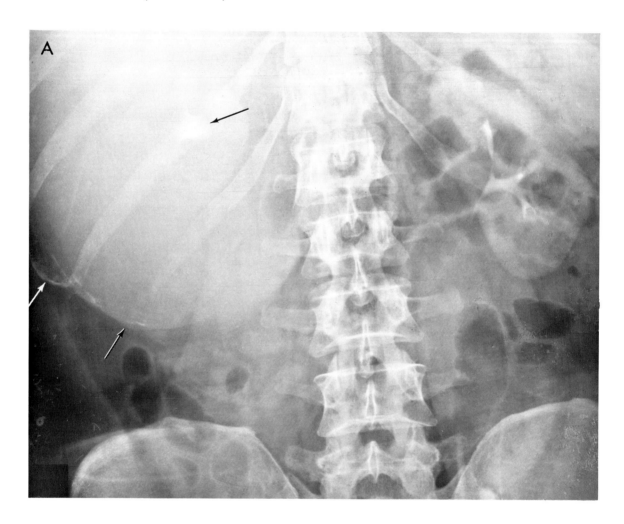

B, retrograde aortogram, anteroposterior view: Showing the right renal artery to be displaced upward (**arrow**) by the huge mass and the intrarenal branches displaced and compressed. Some of the branches seem somewhat splayed, but there is no evidence of tumor vasculature. The caliectasis involving the minor calyces of the upper collecting system seen in **A** is seen to better advantage here.

(*Continued* on p. 80.)

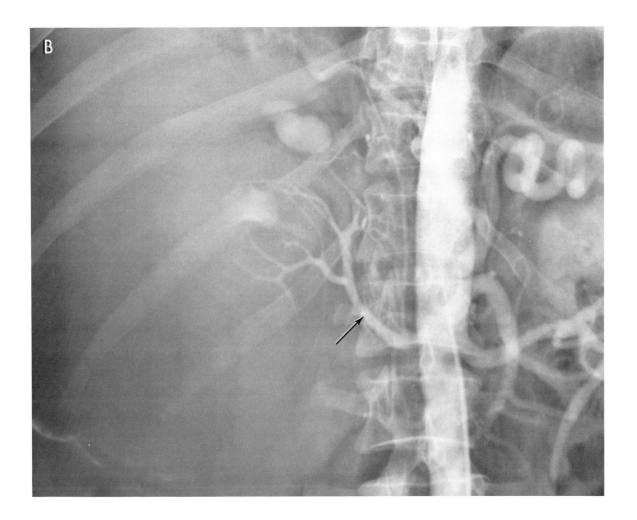

Figure 23 · **Echinococcus Cyst** / **79**

Figure 23 (cont.).—Echinococcus cyst.

C, selective right renal angiogram, late arterial phase, anteroposterior exposure: Revealing a small amount of functioning renal tissue at the upper pole of the large renal mass. The secondary and tertiary branches of the renal artery are thin and attenuated and appear to be draped over the huge mass.

D, inferior venacavogram, right posterior oblique projection: Demonstrating compression of the vena cava as well as compression of the renal pelvis (**y**) and calyces (**x**) by the large mass.

E, surgical specimen: A large echinococcal cyst containing multiple daughter cysts.

A 58-year-old man who was born in Russia but had lived for many years in Turkey and later Germany was hospitalized because of abdominal pain. At nephrectomy, a large echinococcus cyst of the right kidney was found.

Comment: In this case the radiologic findings of a large, calcified, hypovascular mass are not specific and suggest the diagnosis of cystic disease or a necrotic neoplasm. However, with the suggestive history and laboratory findings, the diagnosis of hydatid disease can be made.*

---

* Deliveliotis, A.; Kehayas, P., and Varkarakis, M.: The diagnostic problems of hydatid disease of the kidney, J. Urol. 99:139, 1968.

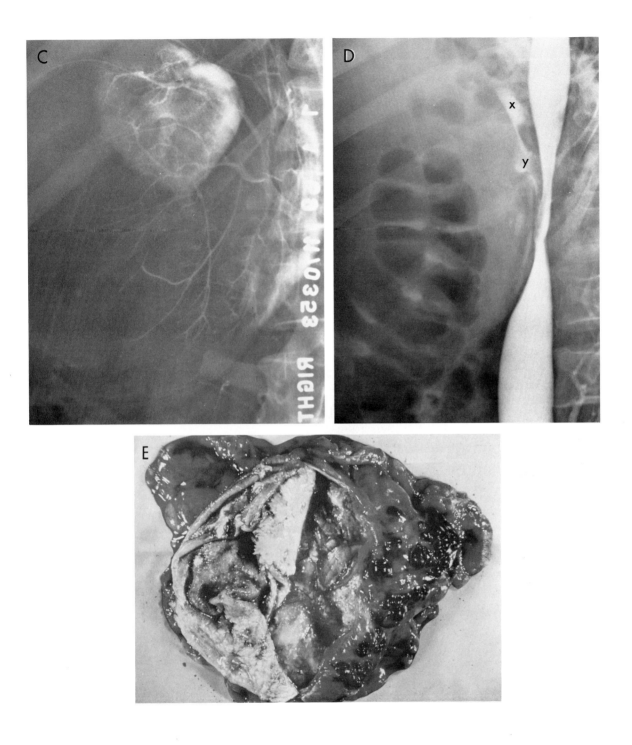

Figure 23 · Echinococcus Cyst / 81

PART 3

Carcinoma of the Kidney Parenchyma

Renal Cell Carcinoma

PRIMARY MALIGNANT TUMORS of the kidney make up 1–3% of all human cancer. Renal cell carcinoma accounts for 80–83% of these tumors. Renal pelvic neoplasms are next most common (7–10%), followed by Wilms' tumor or nephroblastoma (5–6%) and mesenchymal sarcoma (3–4%), discussed in Parts 4 and 7.

HISTOLOGIC AND CLINICAL ASPECTS

Renal cell carcinoma, also called hypernephroma and renal adenocarcinoma, is the commonest primary neoplasm of the kidney. It is the third most common malignant lesion of the urinary tract in men (after prostatic and bladder neoplasms). Renal cell carcinoma is more common in men than in women (3:2) and has its highest incidence at age 50–70, but individuals of all ages can be affected, including children.

The histology of this tumor has been the subject of much debate because of its extreme diversity. It is generally agreed that the tumor arises from the renal tubular epithelium. Rubin's classification is helpful in understanding the various histologic aspects of these lesions. The tumors vary microscopically in: (1) *cell type*, being composed of clear cells or granular cells, or both; (2) *cell morphology*, that is, the state of differentiation or anaplasia, and (3) *cell arrangement*—medullary, tubular, cystic or papillary. Attempts to base prognosis and classification of clinical manifestations on the histologic pattern are not universally accepted, although it is generally agreed that the more anaplastic the cell morphology the worse the prognosis, and it has been said that clear cell tumors have a better prognosis than tumors composed chiefly of granular cells. Prognosis is apparently more accurately evaluated from the presence or absence of capsular invasion and venous infiltration of the tumor.

Metastases from renal cell carcinoma are present at the time of original examination in from 10–40% of reported cases. The lungs are the most common site, metastases from renal cell carcinoma being found in over 50% of one large autopsy series. Lymph nodes, liver and bones are the next most common sites and about equal in involvement, followed by the adrenal, the opposite kidney and the brain.

Renal cell carcinoma most frequently metastasizes via the venous structures. The tumor has a propensity to invade the renal veins and extend up the vena cava, well demonstrated in Figures 62–66. Renal neoplasms also spread via a rich plexus of lymphatics that drain the kidney (Fig. 70) and sometimes by direct extension to adjacent structures (Fig. 56).

The clinical symptomatology associated with renal cell carcinoma is varied, leading to a description of this neoplasm as the "great imitator." This is because the tumor not infrequently is first manifested by symptoms caused by its metastases and because the lesion itself is associated with a number of unusual signs and symptoms. Among the more common ones are hematuria, pain, mass, fever, weight loss, edema of the lower extremities (due to caval obstruction, Fig. 66), gastrointestinal symptoms, hypertension (Figs. 57 and 58), varicocele, polycythemia and anemia. On the other hand, renal cell carcinoma may be totally asymptomatic. In one series 33% of patients did not have urologic symptoms; in another series 40% did not have hematuria. The so-called clinical triad of hematuria, pain and mass is relatively rare, occurring in only 10–15% of cases.

The overall five year survival of patients with renal cell carcinoma is 40–50%. The most important factor in prognosis (if patients who have metastases at the time of diagnosis are excluded) is involvement of the renal vein. The five year survival is below 30% in patients with tumor invasion of the renal vein and over 50% in patients in whom the renal vein is clear.

RADIOLOGIC DIAGNOSIS

The radiologic techniques used to diagnose renal tumors are outlined in Part 1. Here we will summarize the more important radiologic findings in renal cell carcinoma and attempt to demonstrate these signs and manifestations in the following illustrations and comments.

UROGRAPHY.—Renal cell carcinoma can present urographically (and pyelographically) in a number of ways. When presenting as a renal mass, it may cause a bulge in the kidney outline, usually with an associated calyceal deformity. If, however, the lesion grows outward from the cortex of the kidney, calyceal deformity is not present. For this reason it is important to examine the complete contour of the kidney on urography if a peripheral lesion is not to be missed. If the tumor is intrarenal, considerable distortion of the collecting system or obstruction of a calyceal group may occur. In this instance the renal mass is readily discerned. Figure 24 depicts a number of possible urographic appearances associated with renal tumors. Occasionally, the renal pelvis and calyces are invaded and destroyed by extension of the tumor into these areas. This appearance associated with a renal mass indicates renal malignancy, although infection (abscess, tuberculosis) could give a similar picture.

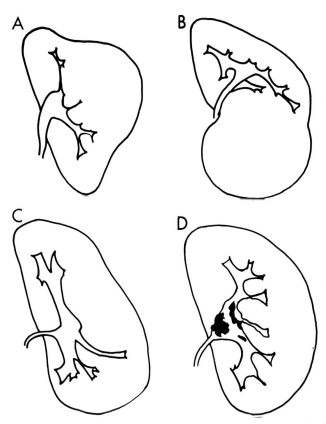

Figure 24.—Common urographic appearances of kidneys involved by tumors. **A,** bulge in the middle pole of the kidney associated with calyceal deformity; **B,** polar enlargement with crowding of calyces; **C,** calyceal deformity without significant kidney contour change; **D,** tumor of renal pelvis.

Another manifestation of renal cell carcinoma may be nonvisualization of the kidney on urography. This may be due to obstruction of the renal vein by tumor, to extension of tumor into the renal pelvis with hydronephrosis or to total replacement of kidney by neoplasm. These possibilities are best studied by retrograde pyelography. On the other hand, tumors confined to the parenchyma presenting as typical masses rarely require retrograde pyelography for diagnosis as this modality will not add further information in this instance. The urographic demonstration of a renal mass requires the use of nephrotomography or renal angiography for further diagnosis since in most cases carcinoma, renal cyst and various pseudotumors of the parenchyma give an identical pattern.

In summary then, urography is the basic screening procedure for renal carcinoma. If the mass contains calcium (see Fig. 25) or invades and destroys calyceal structures, malignancy is strongly suspected. Otherwise,

Figure 24 · Clinical and Radiographic Characteristics / 87

nephrotomography or renal angiography or both are necessary for diagnosis. If the kidney is not visualized on urography, retrograde pyelography will be helpful prior to angiography.

NEPHROTOMOGRAPHY.—The technique of nephrotomography is described in Part 1 and the nephrotomographic picture of cystic disease is demonstrated in Figures 3–7. The findings in renal carcinoma are depicted in Figures 27–29. It is imperative to emphasize that this procedure should be performed and interpreted with utmost care. *All* criteria necessary for a radiologic diagnosis must be present. The major role of nephrotomography is to confirm the presence of a mass suggested on routine urography and to distinguish between simple benign cysts and other lesions. A mass which does not fulfill all the criteria of a simple benign cyst is considered carcinoma until proved otherwise. Nephrotomography generally will not distinguish abscess, granulomas and hematomas from carcinoma.

RENAL ANGIOGRAPHY.—This has become a routine part of the study of renal carcinoma. Figures 30–73 depict various angiographic manifestations of renal cell carcinoma. The great majority of malignancies are readily diagnosed by aortography or selective renal angiography or both. We have included, however, a large number of hypovascular and avascular lesions since these are particularly difficult to diagnose correctly and therefore should be emphasized.

In a study of 100 renal cell carcinomas, Watson *et al.* found that 62 were exceedingly vascular, 16 were moderately vascular, 16 showed minimal vascularity and 6 were avascular. Similar percentages were noted in 80 tumors studied by Boijsen and Folin. This means that over 75% of renal carcinomas are quite vascular and can easily be diagnosed by flush aortography and approximately 95% by selective angiography. Tumor vessels can occasionally be seen only on the *selective* angiogram while not visualized on the aortic flush. The need for careful selective studies is thus emphasized.

The 5% of renal cell carcinomas which have been described as avascular require further comment. These malignancies are really not totally avascular; they are fed by vessels which may be too small to be seen by routine angiography. Therefore the use of other modalities to help evaluate these difficult lesions is necessary, such as epinephrine angiography (Fig. 43), magnification angiography (Fig. 45) and nephrotomography or angiotomography. It is believed that with the utilization of these complementary procedures, the so-called avascular lesions, often misdiagnosed in the past, can be correctly evaluated in such cases.

The diagnosis for a small percentage of renal masses (usually of the hypovascular group) occasionally must be indefinite, such as "a surgical lesion," or "not a benign cyst," or "carcinoma to be ruled out." Since a number of pseudotumors (Part 6) as well as benign lesions can mimic the angiographic findings of malignancy, exploratory surgery or pathologic biopsy is necessary.

Attempts to correlate the angiographic appearance (degree of vascularity) with the histology have had only limited success. Apparently, well-differentiated papillary-tubular renal carcinomas tend to be hypovascular or avascular. Necrotic and cystic lesions also fall in the hypovascular or avascular group. Such lesions are better studied by nephrotomography. The tumors that are hypervascular are usually clear cell carcinomas, but granular cell and mixed tumors may be vascular. Correlation of angiography with histology has not been consistent nor is it clinically important.

A valuable asset of angiography is the outlining of vascular anatomy and extent of the tumor for the surgeon preoperatively. This has assured safe nephrectomy and improved treatment planning. Unusual blood supply to renal carcinomas is accurately outlined (Figs. 32–34, 53–55 and 57) and the extent of the tumor can be determined (Figs. 46, 56, 62–66, 69 and 70). Also, renal angiography has been utilized instead of histologic biopsy in some cases to diagnose renal malignancy and for planning nonsurgical treatment (Figs. 71 and 72). Other aspects of angiography in renal carcinoma are covered in the comments on the following illustrated cases.

BIBLIOGRAPHY

Bennington, J. L., and Kradjian, R. M.: *Renal Carcinoma* (Philadelphia: W. B. Saunders Company, 1967).

Boijsen, E., and Folin, J.: Angiography in the diagnosis of renal carcinoma, Radiologe 1:173, 1961.

Carter, R. L.: The pathology of renal cancer, J.A.M.A. 204:129, 1968.

Evans, J. A.: The accuracy of diagnostic radiology, arteriography and nephrotomography, J.A.M.A. 204:131, 1968.

Folin, J.: Angiography in renal tumors: Its value in diagnosis & differential diagnosis as a complement to conventional methods, Acta Radiol. (Diag.), supp. 267, 1967.

Grabstald, H.: Renal cell carcinoma: Parts I, II and III, New York J. Med. 64:2539, 2658 and 2771, 1964.

Grabstald, H.: Extent of nephrectomy for renal cell cancer, J.A.M.A. 204:135, 1968.

Gregg, D.: Renal and suprarenal tumours in adults, Brit. J. Radiol. 37:128, 1964.

Lucké, B., and Schlumberger, H. G.: "Tumors of the Kidney, Renal Pelvis and Ureter"; Sec. VIII, Fasc. 30 of Armed Forces Institute of Pathology *Atlas of Tumor Pathology* (Washington, D.C.: 1957).

Rubin, P.: Cancer of the urogenital tract: Kidney; Localized renal adenocarcinoma, J.A.M.A. 204:127, 1968.

Watson, R. C.; Fleming, R. J., and Evans, J. A.: Arteriography in the diagnosis of renal carcinoma: Review of 100 cases, Radiology 91:888, 1968.

Weiss, R. M.; Becker, J. A.; Davidson, A. J., and Lytton, B.: Angiographic appearance of renal papillary-tubular adenocarcinomas, J. Urol. 102:661, 1969.

Figure 25.—Calcification in renal cell carcinoma.

Intravenous urogram, anteroposterior projection: Revealing a large mass which involves the lower half of the right kidney and distorts the lower pole calyces and ureteropelvic junction (**arrows**). Flecks of calcium and curvilinear calcification are associated with the mass (**x**).

A 42-year-old man with a recent history of hepatitis entered the hospital because of right upper quadrant discomfort. A cholecystogram revealed a normal gallbladder and also a right upper quadrant mass within which calcific deposits were seen. A right nephrectomy was performed for renal cell carcinoma. The specimen consisted of a large, partially necrotic renal cell carcinoma, containing calcification in the necrotic portions.

Comment: Calcification is a comparatively common finding in renal carcinomas. In a review of a number of series of primary renal neoplasms, roentgenographic evidence of calcification was noted in 15–35%.* The calcium deposits occur mainly in areas of hemorrhage or necrosis. The calcifications usually appear in the form of flecks or stippled densities but occasionally may be linear and ringlike. If a renal mass contains this type of irregular, stippled calcification, benign cyst can be excluded and a solid tumor diagnosed.

---

* Phillips, T. L.; Chin, F. G., and Palubinskas, A. J.: Calcification in renal masses, Radiology 80:786, 1963.

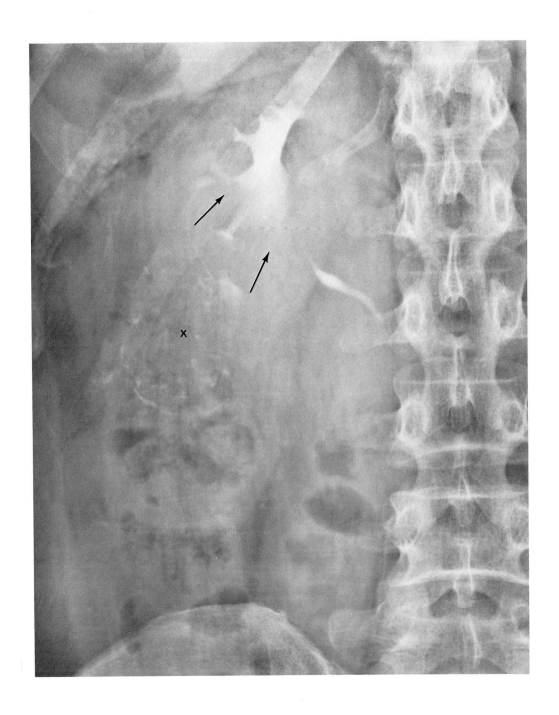

Figure 25 · Calcification in Carcinoma / 91

Figure 26.—Renal cell carcinoma with calcification.

A, intravenous urogram, anteroposterior projection: Showing a rather large, irregularly calcified mass associated with the upper lateral pole of the right kidney and having little effect on the calyceal structures.

B, selective right renal angiogram, right posterior oblique projection: Revealing that the superior capsular artery is slightly dilated and, in the region of the calcified mass it gives off of, a number of small irregular tortuous vessels (**upper arrows**). A few small irregular perforating vessels extend into the mass (**lower arrow**). Some of the small intrarenal branches in the area of the mass are dilated and tortuous. The renal cortex is poorly defined in the area of the tumor, which is situated mostly on the surface of the kidney and extending into the perirenal space.

A woman of 35 had been known to have right upper quadrant calcification for eight years before hospitalization. She had no urinary tract symptoms until two years before admission, when she began to have episodes of right flank pain. Results of urine examination were unremarkable. A right nephrectomy was performed for renal cell carcinoma of the papillary type. Grossly, the tumor was partially cystic and there were areas of organized hematoma.

Comment: Renal carcinoma can be an indolent neoplasm, remaining relatively unchanged for a long period. In this case, the right upper abdominal calcification had been present at least eight years. An apparently unchanged upper abdominal calcified mass in a young person is not usually associated with the diagnosis of renal carcinoma. We have seen a few such patients who have been followed for years without the correct diagnosis being suspected. A renal mass which contains calcium must be considered a malignant lesion until proved otherwise!

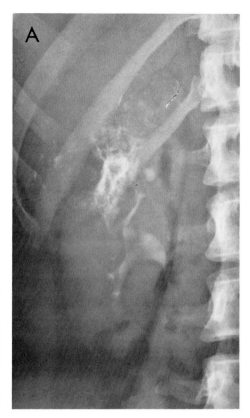

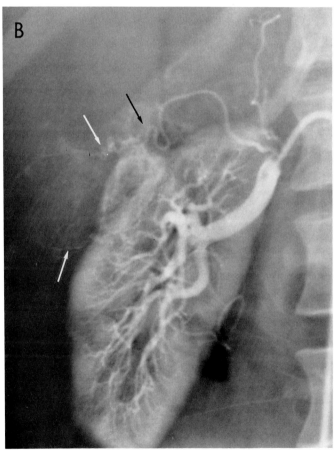

Figure 26 · Calcification in Carcinoma / 93

Figure 27.—Renal cell carcinoma diagnosed by nephrotomography.

A, intravenous aortogram, capillary phase, anteroposterior projection: An example of the original technique of nephrotomography, composed of an intravenous aortogram followed by the tomographic "cuts."* This view shows quite graphically the ability of the intravenous aortogram to demonstrate the vascularity of the renal carcinoma.

B, nephrotomogram: Strikingly demonstrating the basic character of this tumor. The mass is slightly lobulated and despite its distinct and sharp margins is of irregular or uneven density with several radiolucent highlights. Of particular diagnostic importance is the poor and ill-defined interface

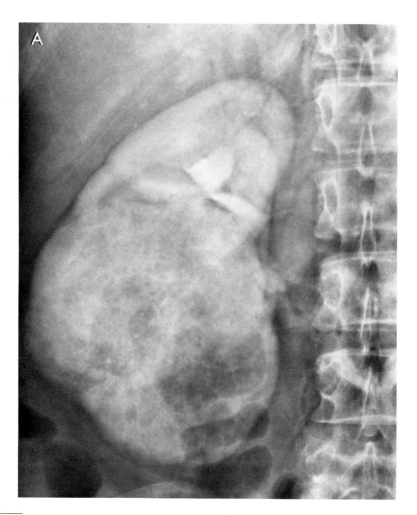

* Evans, J. A.: Nephrotomography in the investigation of renal masses, Radiology 69: 684, 1957.

between mass and normal kidney, in contrast to the sharp, well-defined interface seen in cysts. The lesion is "dense," hence it represents a lesion other than a cyst.

A 49-year-old woman noted a lump in the right flank and entered the hospital for evaluation. There were no symptoms referable to the urinary tract. She underwent a right nephrectomy for a renal cell carcinoma.

Comment: These nephrotomographic findings are classically those of a malignant tumor. The radiologic pathologic anatomy portrayed by this nephrotomogram reflects accurately the gross tumor pathology seen on section of the specimen—a well-circumscribed, partially necrotic renal cell carcinoma.

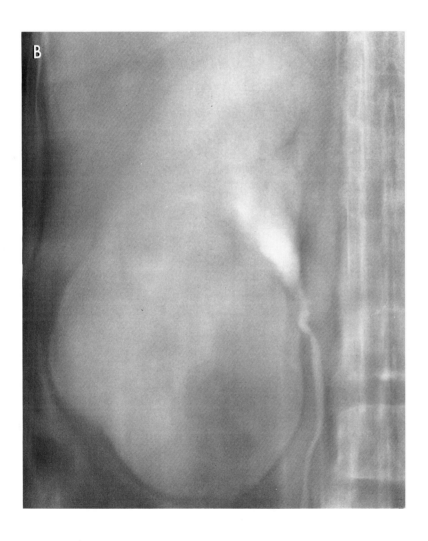

Figure 27 · Carcinoma: Nephrotomograms / 95

Figure 28.—Renal cell carcinoma diagnosed by nephrotomography.

A, intravenous urogram, anteroposterior exposure: Showing a mass occupying the upper and middle poles of the left kidney, with distortion of the collecting system and hydronephrosis of the upper pole calyces.

B, intravenous aortogram, arterial phase, anteroposterior view: Demonstrating the aorta and its branches. The left intrarenal vessels are distorted and stretched (**arrows**), but there are no obvious tumor vessels or tumor stain.

C, nephrotomogram, anteroposterior projection: Showing a large well-defined mass of uneven radiolucency bounded by a thick ragged wall (**arrows**) occupying the upper half of the kidney.

A man of 51 was hospitalized because of painless hematuria. A left nephrectomy was performed for a necrotic renal cell carcinoma.

Comment: The nephrotomographic findings indicate that the lesion is not a simple benign cyst and make the diagnosis of neoplasm almost certain, although renal abscess can have a similar appearance.

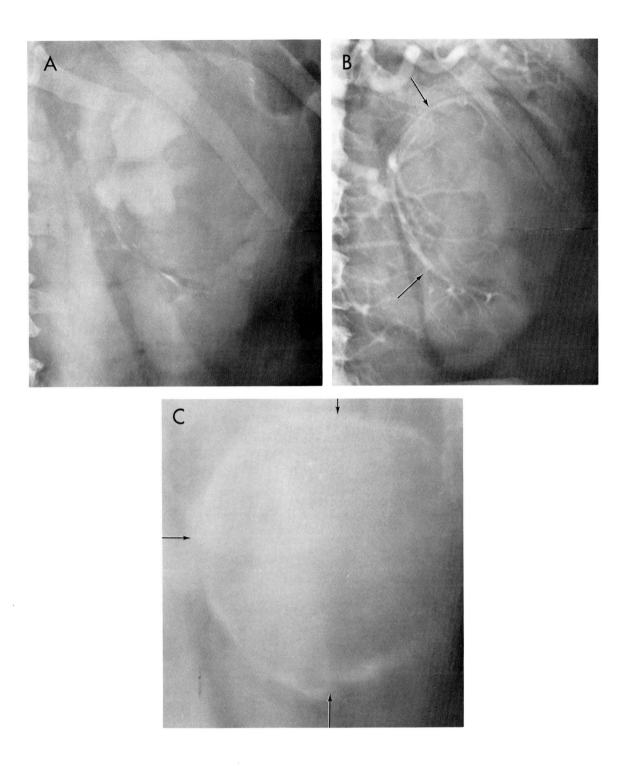

Figure 28 · Carcinoma: Nephrotomograms / 97

Figure 29.—"Thick wall sign" indicating malignant renal tumor.

Nephrotomogram, anteroposterior exposure: Revealing a large, well-marginated, uniformly radiolucent mass involving the upper pole of the left kidney. It might well be mistaken for a benign cyst except for the thick wall (**arrows**). The presence of a thick wall immediately excludes consideration of a benign cyst and should strongly suggest a cystic or necrotic neoplasm. Also delineated is a round mass above the kidney (**x**). This is the pseudo-tumor caused by the fundus of the stomach filled with fluid. Note its continuity with the air-filled antrum of the stomach (**y**).

A 66-year-old woman entered the hospital with hematuria. She had metastatic disease to the bones and lungs, and a biopsy specimen of a bone lesion revealed metastatic renal cell carcinoma.

Comment: An extremely important radiologic finding is demonstrated in this case. In nephrotomography, if a lesion is seen with thick walls, it cannot be considered a simple benign cyst and must be studied further (see Bosniak and Faegenburg below). It might represent a necrotic carcinoma or abscess or possibly an infected cyst.

Figure 29, courtesy of Bosniak, M. A., and Faegenburg, D.: The thick-wall sign: An important finding in nephrotomography, Radiology 84:692, 1965.

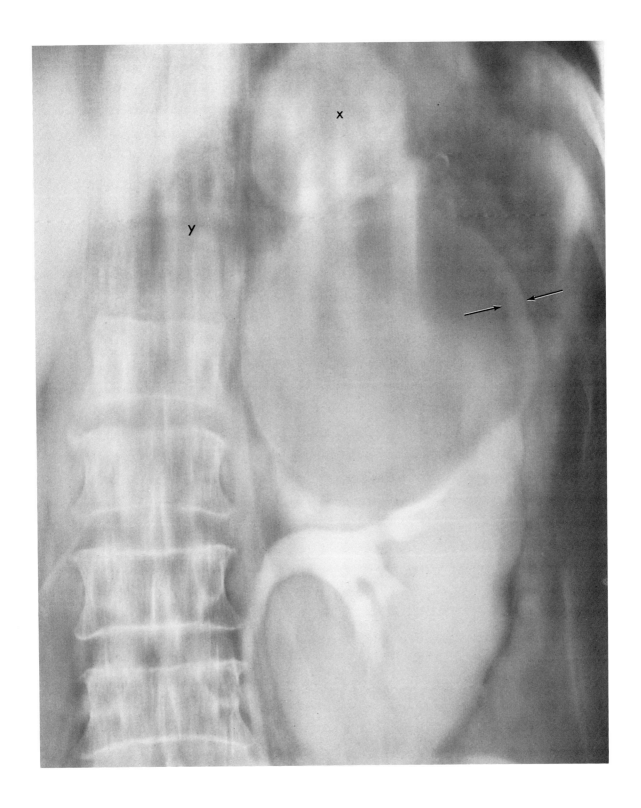

Figure 29 · Carcinoma: Thick Wall Sign / 99

Figure 30.—Large vascular renal cell carcinoma.

    A, intravenous urogram, anteroposterior projection: Showing a large mass (**x**) at the upper pole of the right kidney with distortion of the upper pole calyx (**arrow**).

(*Continued* on p. 104.)

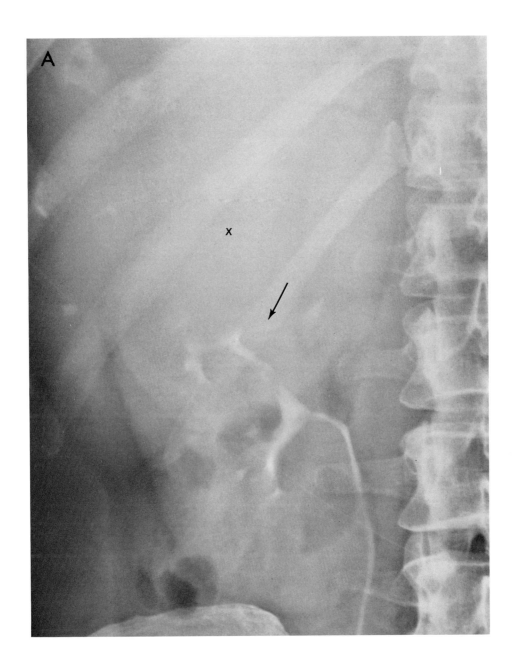

Figure 30 · Large Vascular Carcinoma / 101

Figure 30 (cont.).—Large vascular renal cell carcinoma.

B, selective right renal arteriogram, arterial phase, anteroposterior view: Demonstrating a large vascular neoplasm. Note the tortuous, irregular serpiginous vessels in the neoplasm, which is well demarcated. The lower pole of the kidney is not involved.

C, same study, nephrogram phase: An irregular, blotchy nephrogram, demonstrating areas of increased density and radiolucency. Note filling of the renal vein, indicating its patency (**arrows**).

A woman, age 50, was hospitalized because of right upper quadrant discomfort. A right nephrectomy was performed. Pathologic diagnosis was well-encapsulated renal cell carcinoma. The renal vein was free from tumor.

Comment: This case demonstrates the classic appearance of a vascular renal cell carcinoma. The renal artery and vein and tumor vessels are amply delineated, and the well-marginated encapsulated tumor is clearly defined.

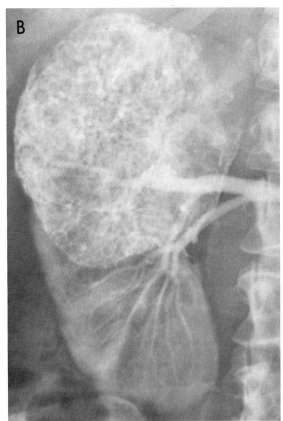

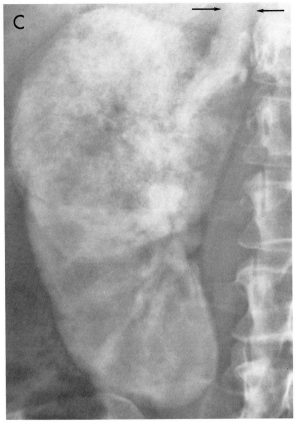

Figure 30 · Large Vascular Carcinoma / 103

Figure 31.—Vascular renal cell carcinoma.

A, right retrograde pyelogram, anteroposterior projection: Demonstrating the presence of a mass involving the lower pole of the right kidney and producing distortion and amputation of calyces.

B, selective right renal arteriogram, arterial phase, right posterior oblique projection: Showing the right renal artery to be enlarged secondary to increased blood flow. The entire intrarenal vasculature is grossly abnormal, presenting as a plethoric mass of tumor vessels. The vessels show marked irregularity, tortuosity and small aneurysmlike dilatations.

C, same study, nephrogram phase: Delineating large distended veins coursing over the upper and lower portions of the renal mass. Within the large renal mass are spotty areas of diminished opacification which probably represent areas of necrosis within the tumor. The main renal vein is seen and appears to be normal (**arrows**).

A man of 74 was hospitalized because of hematuria of four weeks' duration. A right nephrectomy was performed. A large renal cell carcinoma replaced about 95% of the renal parenchyma. Areas of necrosis were common. Numerous veins in the perirenal fat were engorged, and a small secondary branch of the renal vein was involved by tumor. There were multiple adjacent confluent tumor nodules.

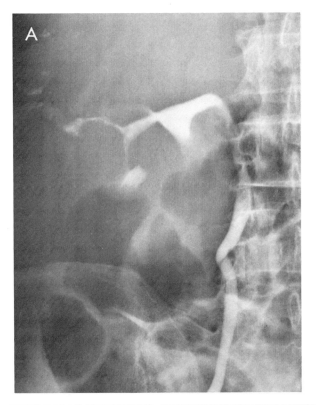

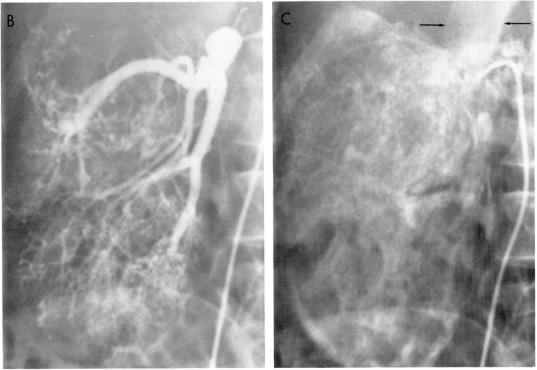

Figure 31 · Vascular Carcinoma / 105

Figure 32.—Huge renal cell carcinoma with hypertrophied capsular artery.

A, intravenous urogram, anteroposterior exposure: Showing a large mass in the upper pole of the right kidney producing calyceal displacement and distortion.

B, selective right renal arteriogram, anteroposterior view: Demonstrating the highly vascular upper pole mass with numerous irregularly dilated and tortuous vessels having the characteristic appearance of neoplastic vessels.

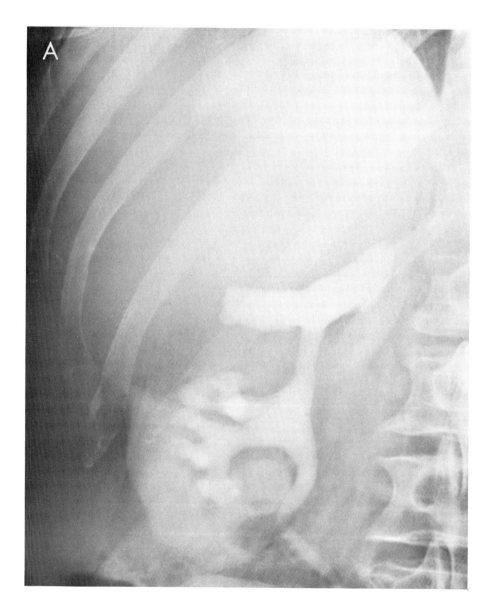

The extent of the lesion to the diaphragm is well shown. The hypertrophied capsular artery outlines and supplies the superior margin of the tumor (**arrows**).

A 70-year-old man was hospitalized because of right upper quadrant discomfort. At right nephrectomy a renal cell carcinoma was removed.

Comment: Capsular arteries frequently hypertrophy to help feed peripherally located lesions (see Figs. 54 and 55). Occasionally they are the main blood supply to peripheral tumors (see Fig. 26, **B**).

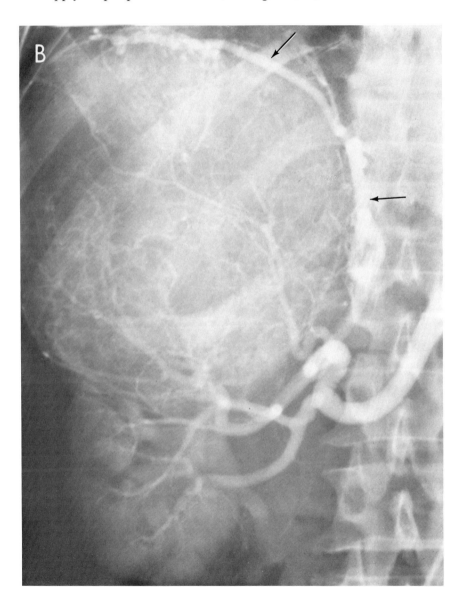

Figure 32 · **Carcinoma with Hypertrophied Capsular Artery** / **107**

Figure 33.—Renal cell carcinoma fed by two renal arteries.

A, intravenous urogram, anteroposterior exposure: Revealing a mass (**x**) in the upper pole of the left kidney that causes calyceal distortion and displacement.

B, nephrotomogram, anteroposterior view: Showing a large, irregularly dense mass (**x**) with thick walls (**arrows**) which involves the upper half of the kidney. The nephrotomographic appearance is characteristic of a malignant neoplasm.

C, and **D,** selective left renal arteriograms, arterial phases, anteroposterior projections: Showing that two renal arteries to the left kidney have been catheterized. A large, highly vascular neoplasm with typical neoplastic vessels is supplied by both arteries. Large capsular arteries supplying the retroperitoneal space are also seen (**C**) (**arrows**).

A man, age 56, was admitted to the hospital because of weight loss, left flank pain and one episode of hematuria. A renal cell carcinoma was removed at surgery.

Comment: Multiple renal arteries to the kidney occur in 15–20% of the population. Usually a neoplasm in such a kidney draws its blood supply from both vessels. Occasionally, however, as shown in Figure 53, the renal neoplasm is supplied by only one of the two arteries.

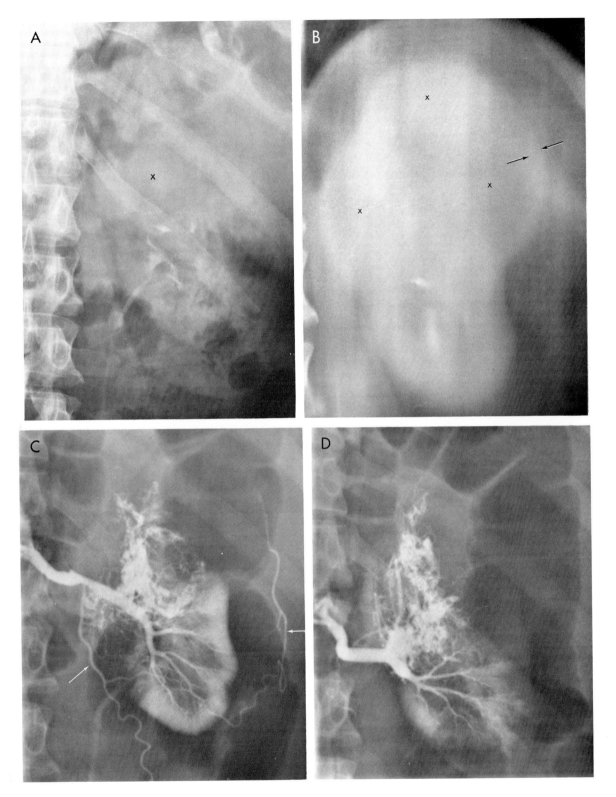

Figure 33 · Carcinoma Fed by Two Renal Arteries / 109

Figure 34.—Renal cell carcinoma with two renal arteries.

A, retrograde pyelogram, anteroposterior view: Demonstrating poor and incomplete filling of the renal pelvis, minimal dilatation of the calyces and the suggestion of a peripelvic mass.

B, aortogram, anteroposterior projection: Delineating two renal arteries (**arrows**) that supply a vascular tumor of the kidney.

C, selective left renal arteriogram of upper vessel, anteroposterior view: Revealing a highly vascular tumor of the kidney with typical tumor vasculature.

D, same study of lower vessel: Showing that the upper pole of the kidney is not involved by neoplasm, but some tumor vasculature is evident in the midpole and lower portion of the kidney (**arrow**).

A 64-year-old man was hospitalized because of gross hematuria. Intravenous urography failed to demonstrate the left kidney. After further studies and radiographic diagnosis, nephrectomy was done. A typical clear cell carcinoma was found, with a tumor thrombus in the renal vein.

Comment: Preoperative anatomic delineation of two renal arteries supplying the neoplasm was of value to the surgeon in the performance of nephrectomy. The finding of tumor thrombus in the renal vein probably explains failure of visualization of the kidney on the intravenous urogram.

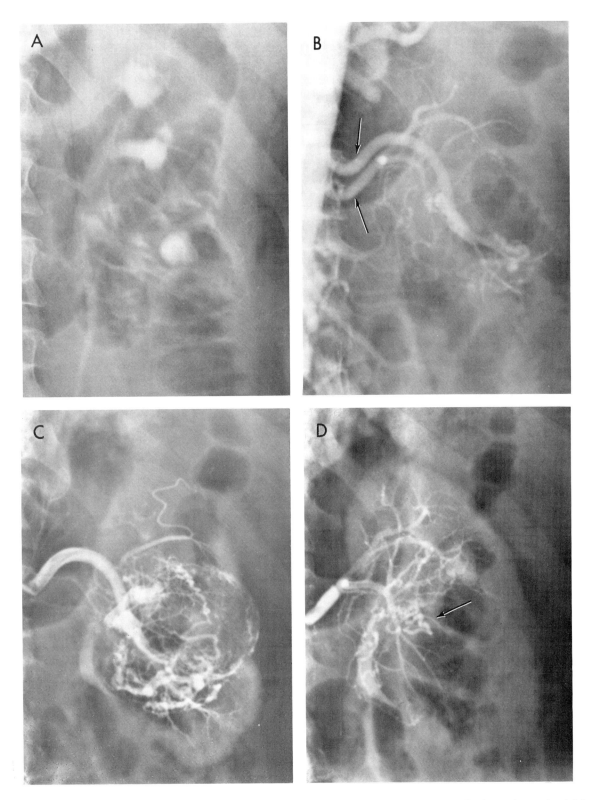

Figure 34 · Carcinoma Fed by Two Renal Arteries / 111

Figure 35.—Huge necrotic hypovascular carcinoma of the kidney.

A, left retrograde pyelogram, anteroposterior view: Revealing a huge mass in the left side of the abdomen displacing the ureter across the midline.

(*Continued* on p. 114.)

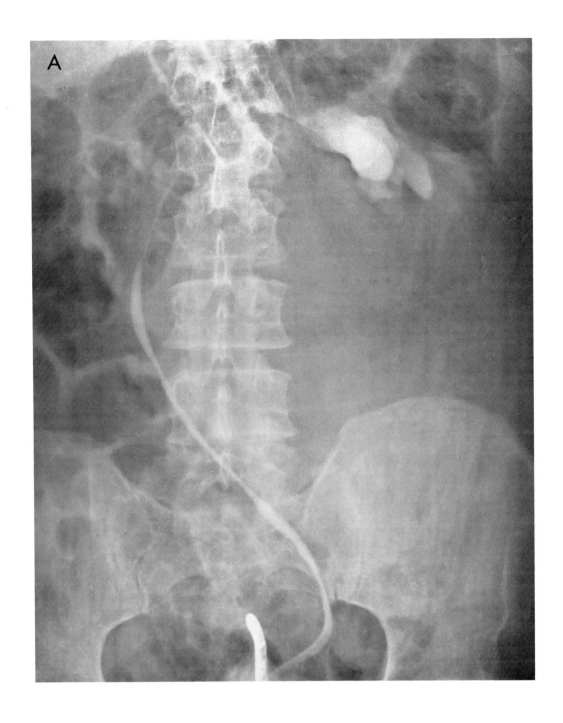

Figure 35 · Necrotic Hypovascular Carcinoma / 113

Figure 35 (cont.).—Huge necrotic hypovascular carcinoma of the kidney.

B, selective left arteriogram, late arterial-capillary phase: Showing a large mass at the lower pole of the kidney. Note numerous perforating vessels extending from the kidney into the mass (**arrows**). Density (**x**) extending from the kidney at the hilus is the renal pelvis filled with contrast medium displaced over the large mass.

C, pathologic specimen: Showing a huge carcinoma arising from the lower pole of the kidney and filled with necrotic, hemorrhagic tissue. The lesion ruptured when it was removed. Diagnosis was renal cell carcinoma.

A man of 66 was hospitalized because a left-sided abdominal mass, known to be present for four years, had recently increased in size. Intravenous urography disclosed elevation of the kidney and displacement of the left ureter to the midline by a huge mass in the left flank.

Comment: Two points are important in this case. (1) The indolent nature of cystic carcinoma of the kidney is documented, the mass having been present for four years. Recent enlargement was probably due to hemorrhage into the tumor. (2) The importance of selective renal arteriography for accurate diagnosis is demonstrated. In the flush (midstream) aortic injection, the small vessels supplying the neoplasm seen in **B** were not appreciated. They could only be seen on the selective study. Some observers* question the accuracy of angiography in renal mass lesions. The accuracy of angiography cannot be judged from studies based on translumbar, midstream aortograms without selective angiography.

---

* Uson, A. C.; Melicow, M. M., and Lattimer, J. K.: Is renal arteriography (aortography) a reliable test in the differential diagnosis between kidney cysts and neoplasms? J. Urol. 89: 554, 1963.

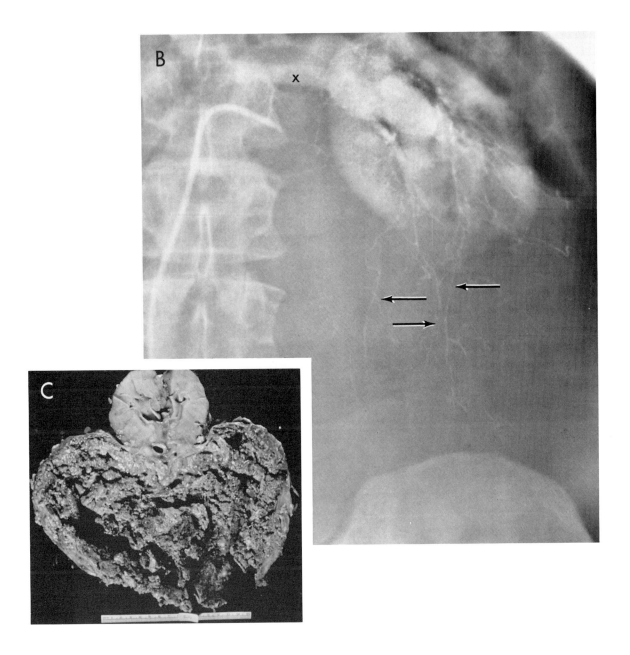

Figure 35 · Necrotic Hypovascular Carcinoma / 115

Figure 36.—Hypovascular renal cell carcinoma of the left kidney.

A, intravenous urogram, anteroposterior view: Revealing a large mass protruding from the lower pole of the left kidney (**arrows**).

(*Continued* on p. 119.)

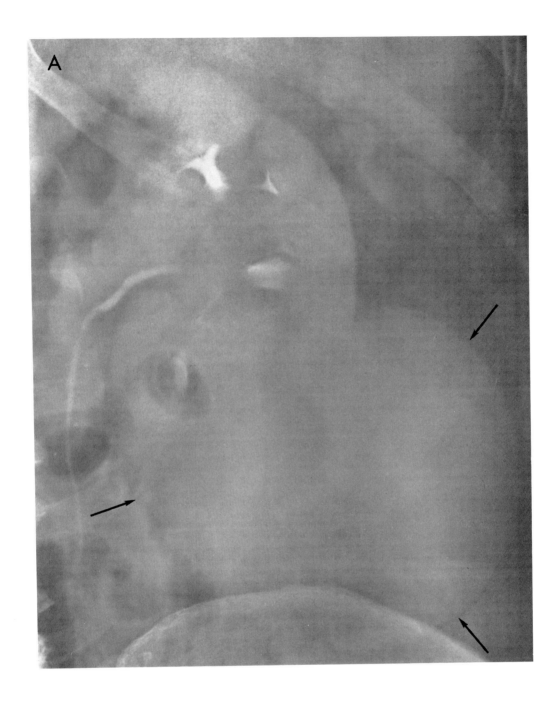

Figure 36 · Necrotic Hypovascular Carcinoma / 117

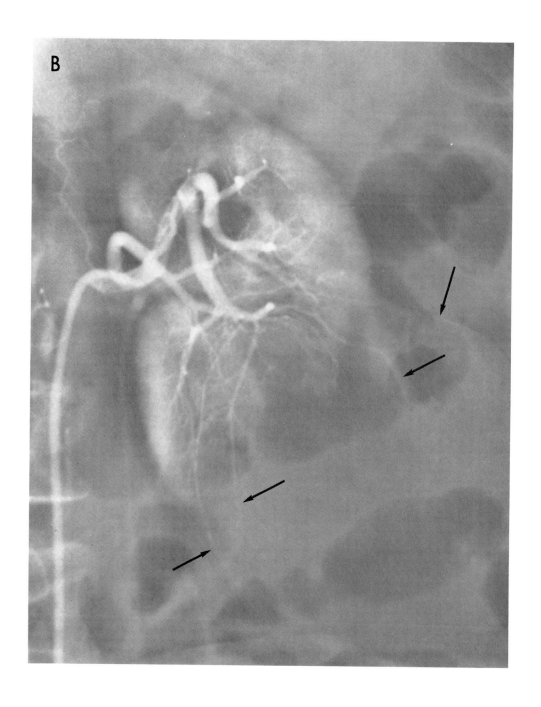

Figure 36 (cont.).—Hypovascular renal cell carcinoma of the left kidney.

B, selective left renal arteriogram, anteroposterior view: Delineating normal intrarenal vessels, but a number of slightly hypertrophied vessels extend outside of the kidney to supply the lesion (**arrows**). This rules out a simple benign cyst and indicates a diagnosis of malignant tumor or possibly a renal abscess.

C, pathologic specimen: A large, solid, avascular clear cell carcinoma.

A man of 66 was hospitalized because of prostatic enlargement.

Comment: The arteriogram established the diagnosis of malignancy in this case. The vessels extending out of the kidney to supply the renal mass indicate that the lesion is not a simple benign cyst. Arteries of this size will not feed the wall of simple nonneoplastic lesions, so the diagnosis must be a malignancy (or abscess). If accurate diagnosis of such hypovascular neoplasms is to be made, detailed selective angiograms must be obtained.

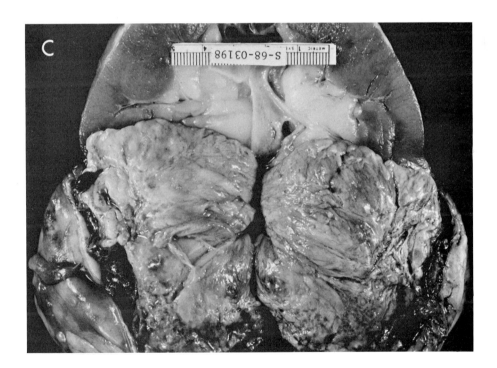

Figure 36 · Necrotic Hypovascular Carcinoma / 119

Figure 37.—Hypovascular carcinoma of the left kidney.

A, selective left renal arteriogram, arterial phase, anteroposterior projection: Showing a mass at the lower pole of the kidney supplied by perforating vessels from the kidney. Some irregular-appearing vessels supply the capsule of the cystic neoplasm (**arrows**).

B, same study, nephrogram phase: Showing the mass to be relatively smooth and radiolucent but surrounded by a thick wall (**arrows**) characteristic of a necrotic or cystic neoplasm.

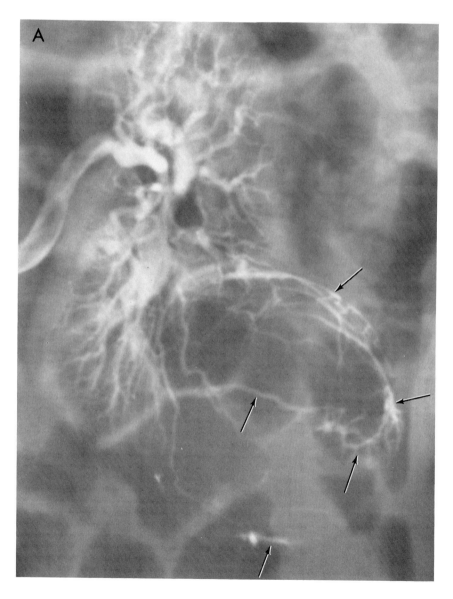

A 56-year-old man was hospitalized because of hematuria and persistent fever. Intravenous urography revealed a mass at the lower pole of the left kidney. At left nephrectomy a cystic mass was found, the cavity of which was glistening and smooth. Microscopic section, however, disclosed a renal cell carcinoma in the wall.

Comment: The findings in this case are quite characteristic of a cystic malignancy of the kidney.

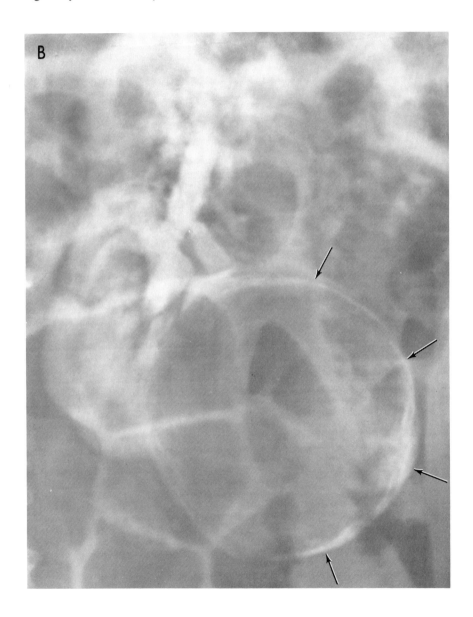

Figure 37 · Hypovascular Carcinoma: Thick Wall / 121

Figure 38.—Hypovascular renal cell carcinoma with extension into the renal pelvis.

A, intravenous urogram, anteroposterior exposure: Revealing a duplicated collecting system in the right kidney. In the lower collecting system, caliectasis of midpole and lower pole calyces are seen; the renal pelvis is incompletely visualized. The upper collecting system is normal.

B, right retrograde pyelogram of inferior collecting system, anteroposterior projection: Demonstrating a large ovoid filling defect in the renal pelvis (**x**).

(*Continued* on p. 124.)

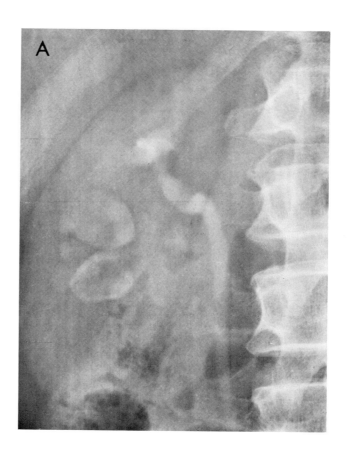

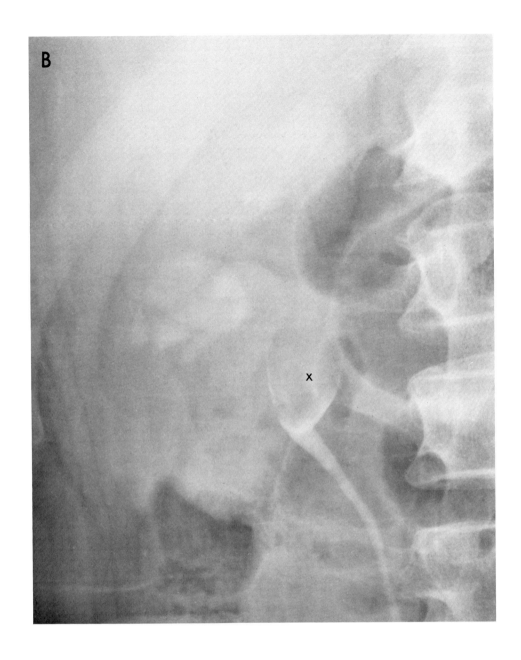

Figure 38 · Hypovascular Carcinoma with Extension / 123

Figure 38 (cont.).—Hypovascular renal cell carcinoma with extension into the renal pelvis.

C, selective right renal arteriogram, arterial phase, anteroposterior exposure: Delineating a group of abnormal appearing vessels occupying the lower pole (**arrows**). The intrarenal vessels in the remainder of the kidney are normal. Note the two hydrocalyces in the midportion of the kidney (**x**) filled from a prior injection of contrast medium.

D, same study, nephrogram phase: Showing an irregular radiolucent lesion that involves the lower pole. Within the radiolucent zone can be seen areas of slight tumor blush (**y**). Note also the loss of the usual cortical rim at the lower pole.

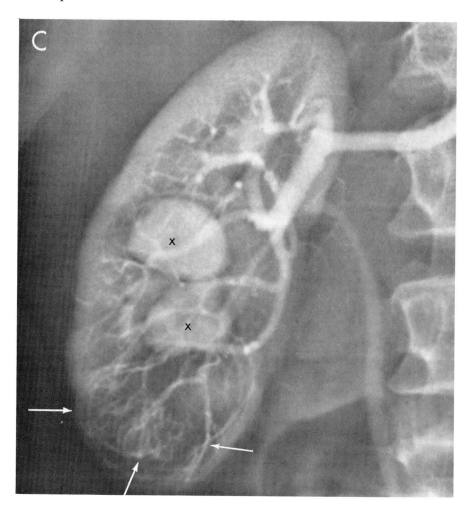

A 50-year-old man was examined because of occasional blood in the urine. A right nephrectomy revealed an 8 cm tumor in the inferior pole of the kidney with strands of tumor projecting into the pelvis which account for the filling defect on pyelography (**B**). The tumor extended to within 1 mm of the cortical margin and into the renal vein.

Comment: The appearance of the smooth, sharply marginated filling defect in the renal pelvis seen in **B** is not unlike that of an impacted stone (radiolucent) or blood clot. The selective arteriogram, however, demonstrates abnormal vasculature in the lower pole of this kidney, and the pooling of contrast medium (tumor stain) in the nephrogram indicates the malignant character of the lesion.

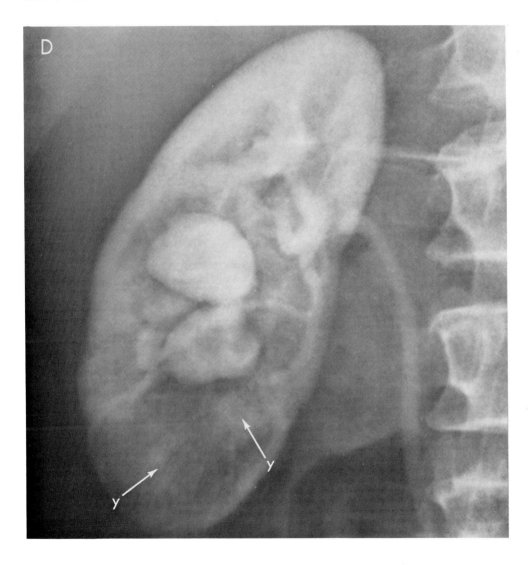

Figure 38 · Hypovascular Carcinoma with Extension / 125

Figure 39.—Hypovascular renal cell carcinoma of the left kidney.

A, intravenous urogram, anteroposterior projection: Showing a 3 cm mass projecting from the lower pole of the left kidney (**x**).

B, nephrotomogram, anteroposterior exposure: Disclosing a lesion (**x**) whose appearance is strikingly similar to that of a simple benign cyst except that it is slightly more "dense" than expected for a cyst.

(*Continued* on p. 128.)

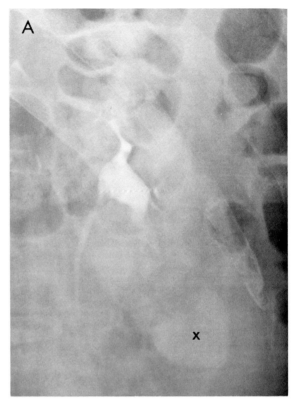

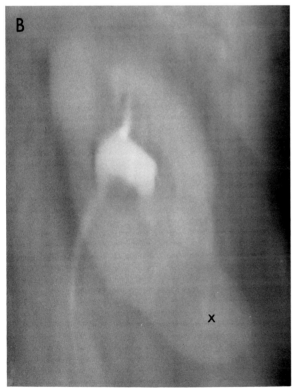

Figure 39 · Hypovascular Carcinoma / 127

Figure 39 (cont.).—Hypovascular renal cell carcinoma of the left kidney.

C, selective left renal arteriogram, arterial phase, anteroposterior view: Delineating a hypovascular mass (**x**) without definite evidence of neoplastic vessels. Note, however, hypertrophy of a perforating capsular artery (**arrow**).

D, same study, early nephrogram phase: Revealing some vascularity in the wall of the lesion as well as some thin tortuous vessels coursing around and over the mass (**arrows**).

During hospital evaluation for prostatism, this man of 69 was found to have an abnormal pyelogram. After further studies, surgery revealed a cystic tumor with prominent vessels on its surface and a smooth white wall attached to the lower pole of the kidney.

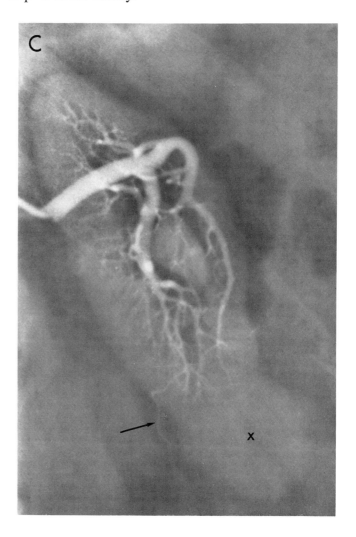

Figure 39 (cont.).—Hypovascular renal cell carcinoma of the left kidney.

Comment: The angiographic findings indicate that the lesion represents something other than a simple benign renal cyst. A similar angiographic appearance can be produced by renal abscess, infected cyst, benign tumor and necrotic neoplasm. It is important, therefore, when the angiographic findings do not clearly reflect those of a simple benign cyst that the patient be explored.

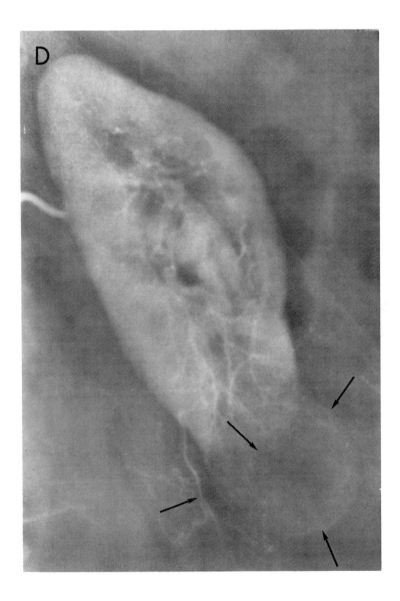

Figure 39 · Hypovascular Carcinoma / 129

Figure 40.—Avascular renal cell carcinoma.

A, right retrograde pyelogram, anteroposterior view: Demonstrating a mass on the anterolateral aspect of the right kidney (**x**) compressing the calyces and renal pelvis (**arrow**). This configuration had not been present on examination seven months earlier.

B, selective right renal arteriogram, arterial phase, anteroposterior exposure: Showing well-filled renal arteries with no intrinsic abnormality. The intrarenal arteries are, however, compressed and displaced by a large mass which appears to be extrarenal.

C, same study, arterial phase, right posterior oblique projection: Showing the extrarenal nature of the mass.

D, same study, nephrogram phase, anteroposterior view: Disclosing no tumor vessels or tumor stain. However, the outer margin of the kidney is not sharp, and the nephrogram in the upper medial margin is incomplete.

A month before these studies a woman of 75 had a sharp right flank pain that persisted intermittently as a dull aching pain. Right oophorectomy had been performed for carcinoma nine months previously. Surgery after the studies shown here revealed an enlarged indurated kidney due to subcapsular hemorrhage with an underlying 4.5 cm anaplastic clear cell carcinoma.

Comment: The conventional urographic examination and also angiography were highly suggestive of extrarenal tumor. Preoperative diagnoses included metastasis to the surface of the kidney secondary to the previously removed ovarian tumor, sarcoma of the renal capsule and subcapsular hematoma. Despite the technically excellent angiographic study, no definite evidence of tumor vascularity was noted. Unfortunately, an epinephrine study was not obtained. Although the angiogram did not establish that the lesion was a primary malignancy of the kidney, it did demonstrate that a surgical lesion of the kidney was present.

This case also demonstrates a rare presentation of renal cortical neoplasm—spontaneous renal hematoma. This bleeding (occurring outside of the collecting system) may be intrarenal or perirenal but is often subcapsular, as in this case. Spontaneous subcapsular hematoma in the absence of anticoagulation therapy, trauma or periarteritis nodosa should make one think of an underlying neoplasm, although spontaneous idiopathic hematoma can occur.

Figure 40, courtesy of Watson, R. C.; Fleming, R. J., and Evans, J. A.: Arteriography in the diagnosis of renal carcinoma: Review of 100 cases, Radiology 91:888, 1968.

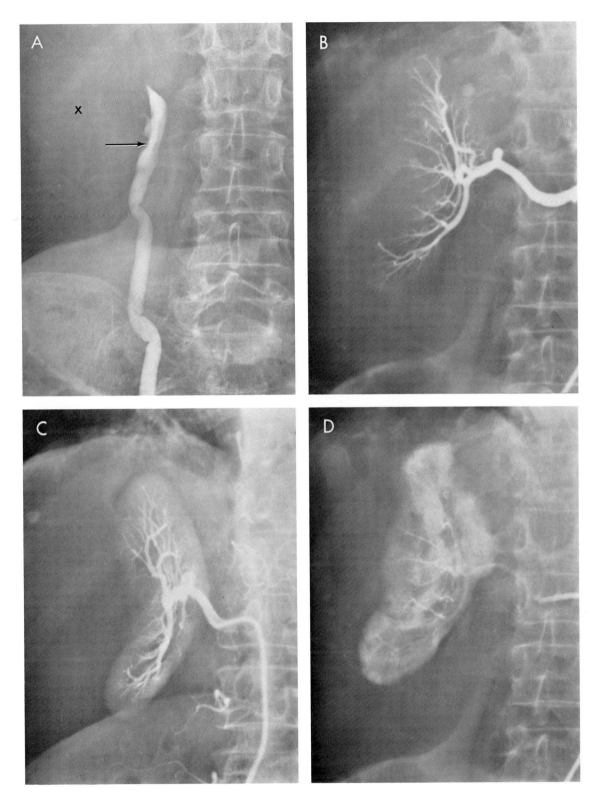

Figure 40 · Avascular Carcinoma / 131

Figure 41.—"Avascular" renal cell carcinoma.

A, selective right renal arteriogram, arterial phase, anteroposterior exposure: Showing a mass in the center of the kidney that displaces the intrarenal branches (**arrows**). The lesion is apparently avascular although some suspicious areas are seen at (**z**). Note the large capsular-inferior adrenal artery (**x**). The kidney has an almost horizontal appearance.

B, same study, nephrogram phase: Demonstrating a radiolucent mass in the center of the kidney. The lesion has a peculiar irregular shape and is not smooth, round and regular as would be expected if it were an intrarenal benign cyst. Slow flow in vessels around the mass (**arrow**) should make one suspicious. Note normal vascularity in the adrenal gland (**y**).

A youth of 20 was hospitalized because of intermittent gross hematuria of three months' duration. Intravenous urography disclosed a right intrarenal

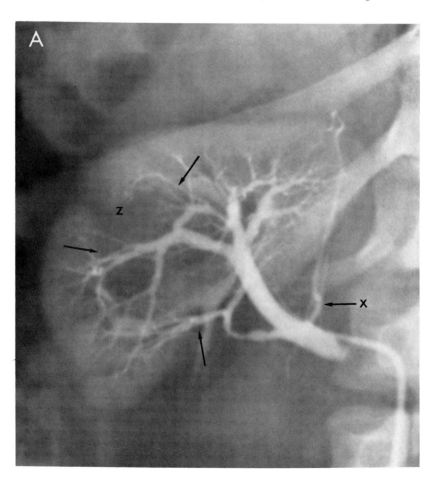

mass. Right nephrectomy was performed for renal cell carcinoma.

Comment: This is an example of an "avascular" carcinoma which can be extremely difficult to diagnose correctly. No definite abnormal vessels are seen (although a few suspicious areas are noted), and the mass could be confused with a benign lesion. However, the irregularity of the contours of the mass might alert one to the fact that a more serious lesion is present. Nephrotomography to delineate the contour of the lesion to better advantage might have been of value, as would the use of epinephrine angiography to bring out tumor vascularity. In any event, the mass is clearly not a benign cyst and therefore must be surgically explored.

Figure 41, courtesy of Watson, R. C.; Fleming, R. J., and Evans, J. A.: Arteriography in the diagnosis of renal carcinoma: Review of 100 cases, Radiology 91:888, 1968.

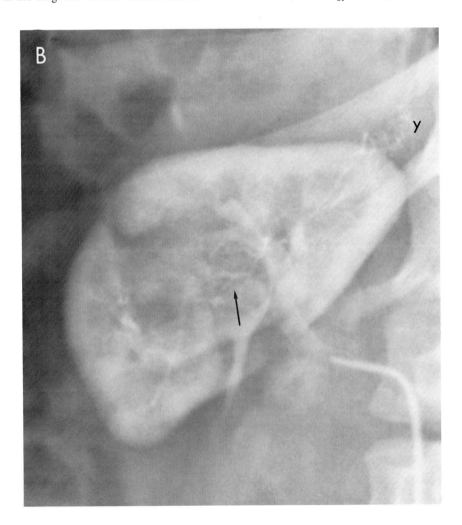

Figure 41 · "Avascular" Carcinoma / 133

Figure 42.—Renal cell carcinoma: epinephrine study.

A, selective left renal arteriogram, anteroposterior exposure: Delineating irregular, tortuous arteries in the upper pole of the kidney (**x**) that are typical of neoplastic vessels.

B, same study after intrarenal introduction of 8 µg of epinephrine: Showing a dramatic increase in the delineation of tumor vessels and clearly indicating the extent of the tumor. Vessels in the remaining portion of the kidney are not filled by contrast medium. Almost all flow to the kidney is being shunted to the tumor.

A 52-year-old woman entered the hospital for evaluation of hypertension. An excretory urogram disclosed an unsuspected mass at the upper pole of the left kidney. A left nephrectomy was performed and a renal cell carcinoma 4.5 cm in diameter was found.

Comment: This case shows graphically the action of epinephrine on renal neoplasms. Epinephrine constricts the normal arteries and therefore restricts flow through them. The drug does not have a similar effect on tumor vessels, so that they stay open and when angiography is performed the contrast medium perfuses the tumor, enhancing visualization. In most cases the technique is not needed to diagnose renal malignancy, but occasionally it can be of great help (see also Figures 44 and 93).

Figure 42, courtesy of Kahn, P. C., and Wise, H. M.: The use of epinephrine in selective angiography of renal masses, J. Urol. 99:133, 1968.

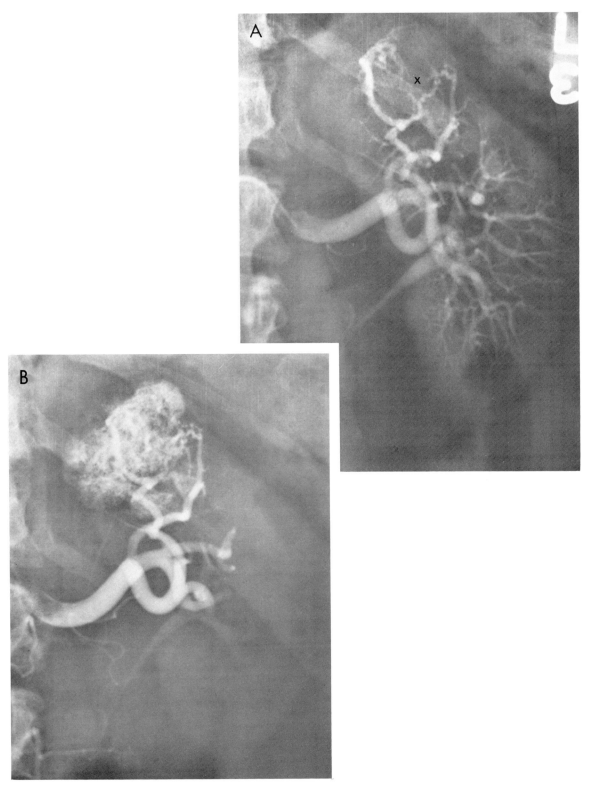

Figure 42 · Carcinoma: Epinephrine Study / 135

Figure 43.—Renal cell carcinoma: epinephrine study.

A, intravenous urogram, anteroposterior projection: Showing a mass in the midportion of the right kidney (**a**).

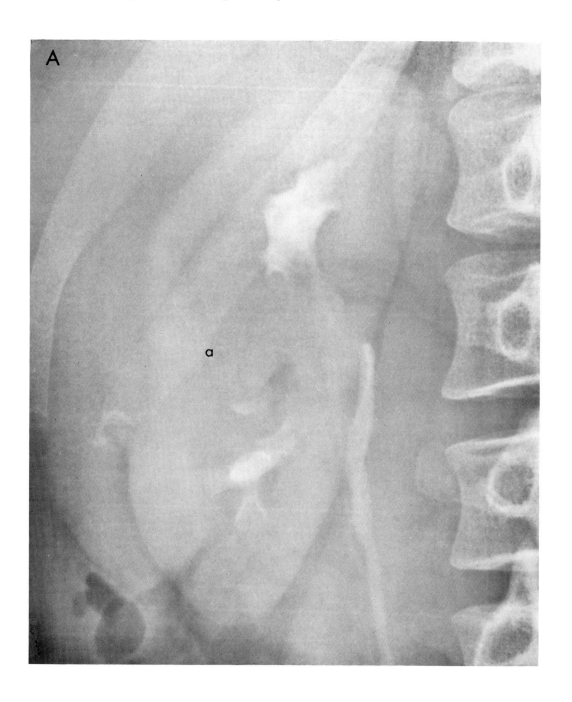

Figure 43 (cont.).—Renal cell carcinoma: epinephrine study.

B, nephrotomogram, anteroposterior view: Demonstrating that the mass is radiolucent but is surrounded by a thick wall (**arrows**), indicating that the lesion is not a benign cyst.

(*Continued* on p. 138.)

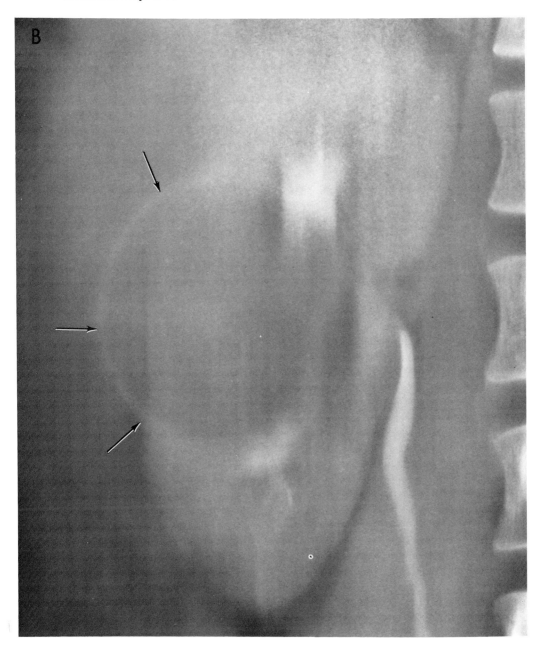

Figure 43 · **Carcinoma: Epinephrine Study / 137**

Figure 43 (cont.).—Renal cell carcinoma: epinephrine study.

C, selective right renal arteriogram, late arterial phase, anteroposterior exposure: Showing abnormal vessels (**arrows**) in the midportion of the kidney that correspond to the renal mass seen in **B** and indicate the malignant nature of the lesion. Considerable filling of the adrenal gland and adrenal vessels (**x**) has also occurred because the renal catheter tip was partly lodged in the inferior adrenal artery, with overfilling of these vessels.

D, selective right renal arteriogram after introduction of 10 μg of epinephrine, early phase: Demonstrating an excellent epinephrine effect, with opacification only of the tumor vessels and no other intrarenal vessels. A catheter is in the unopacified right renal vein.

E, same study after epinephrine introduction, nephrogram phase: Demonstrating a large tumor blush.

The patient, a 31-year-old man, was hospitalized because of hematuria. At right nephrectomy a well-encapsulated lesion was removed.

Comment: On histologic study, the lesion was found to contain cells with clear cytoplasm and small hyperchromatic, often eccentric, nuclei. There was some difference of opinion as to whether this represented adenoma or carcinoma. Histologically, the differentiation between benign adenoma and clear cell renal adenocarcinoma sometimes cannot be made. However, since this lesion measured greater than 3 cm, the diagnosis is considered to be carcinoma. This case also nicely demonstrates the effect of epinephrine on tumor vasculature.

Figure 43, courtesy of Dr. J. A. Becker, State University of New York, Downstate Medical Center, Brooklyn, New York.

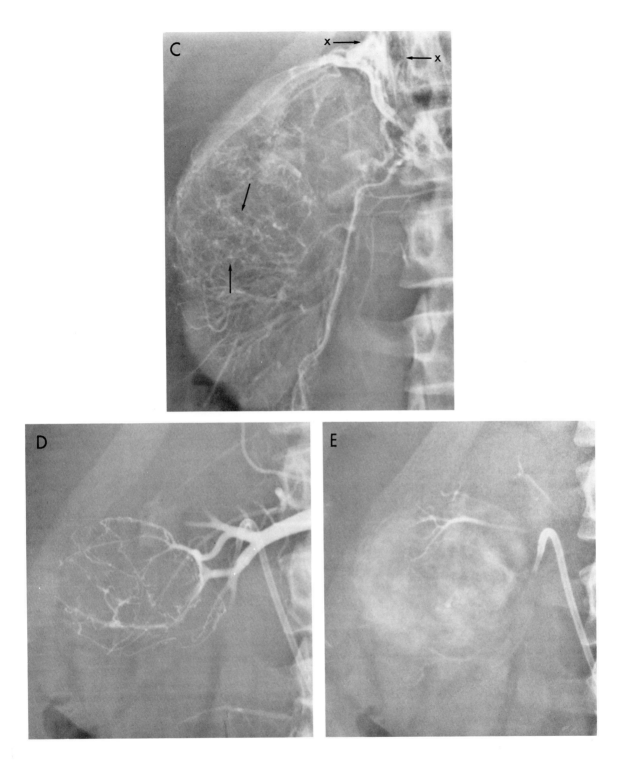

Figure 43 · Carcinoma: Epinephrine Study / 139

Figure 44.—Renal cell carcinoma: epinephrine study.

A, intravenous urogram, anteroposterior projection: Showing a large intrarenal mass that displaces the upper and middle pole calyces of the right kidney and produces mild dilatation of one group of middle calyces. Calcified mesenteric nodes are seen above the right iliac crest.

B, selective right renal arteriogram, anteroposterior view: Demonstrating displacement and deviation of vessels in the upper pole. Some "suspicious" vessels are present (**arrow**).

(*Continued* on p. 142.)

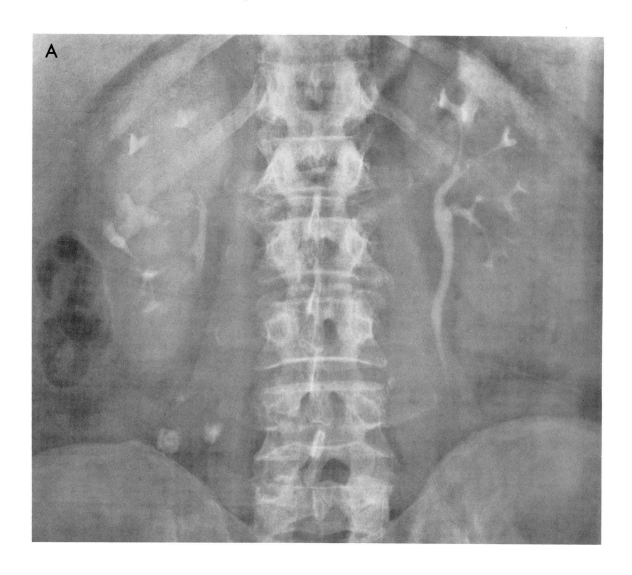

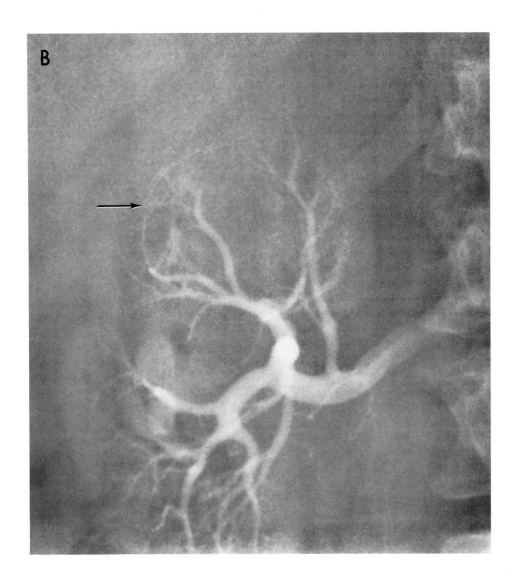

Figure 44 · Carcinoma: Epinephrine Study / 141

Figure 44 (cont.).—Renal cell carcinoma: epinephrine study.

C, same study, after introduction of 8 µg of epinephrine: Indicating that most of the vessels to the right kidney are constricted and therefore not delineated except for the arteries feeding the upper pole. Note the tumor stain (**x**) in this area, indicating malignant neoplasm.

A 56-year-old man was hospitalized because of hematuria. A right nephrectomy revealed a renal cell carcinoma.

Comment: The epinephrine study in this case confirmed the presence of a malignant neoplasm which was barely suggested on the routine study. This is the main value of the epinephrine test—to confirm or deny the malignant nature of a lesion. A positive result such as that obtained here provides confirmation of the suspected diagnosis.

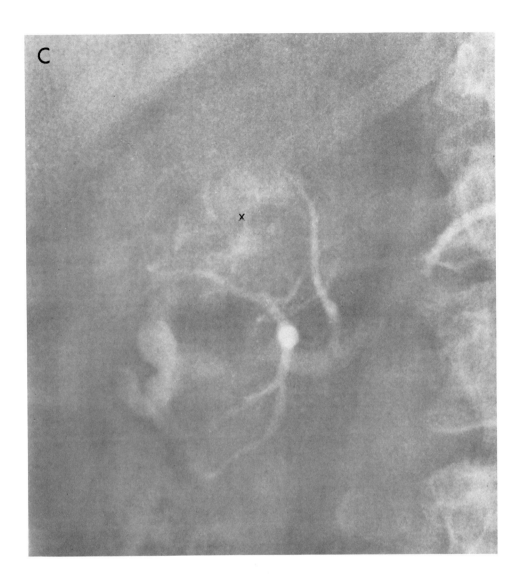

C

Figure 44 · Carcinoma: Epinephrine Study / 143

Figure 45.—Magnification angiography in diagnosis of hypovascular carcinoma.

A, selective left renal arteriogram, nephrogram phase (routine study, no magnification), anteroposterior exposure: Demonstrating a large mass at the lower pole of the left kidney. The lesion is quite hypovascular, but a collection of tumor vessels (**arrow**) is seen, indicating the malignant nature of the lesion.

B, same study, nephrogram phase, with magnification: Allowing better visualization of the hypovascular malignancy than is obtained in **A**. The tumor vessels (**arrow**) are also more clearly seen.

In this patient, nephrectomy was performed for renal cell carcinoma of the left kidney.

Comment: It is difficult to demonstrate the advantages of radiographic magnification photographically. Here, the difference in size between the routine and magnified angiograms has been kept constant throughout the photographic process. Although the conventional angiogram shows all of the abnormalities that the magnified angiogram does, there is no doubt that these findings are more evident on the radiographically magnified film. Theoretically then, in some instances we might expect to see details in the radiographically magnified study that are not seen on the conventional study, thereby improving our diagnostic accuracy in angiography.

Figure 45, courtesy of Dr. H. L. Stein, Manhasset, N.Y.

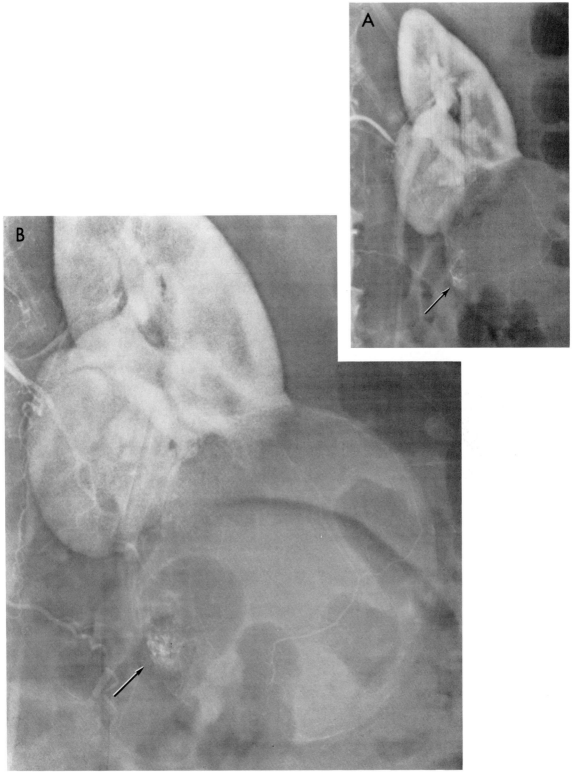

Figure 45 · Carcinoma: Magnification Angiography / 145

Figure 46.—Bilateral renal cell carcinoma.

A, intravenous urogram, anteroposterior projection: Revealing a mass involving the lower pole of the right kidney (**arrows**) that results in deformity and poor filling of the lower pole calyces. The left kidney appears to be normal.

B, retrograde aortogram, anteroposterior exposure: Demonstrating that the mass at the lower pole of the right kidney is a vascular neoplasm (**a**). Unsuspected, however, is the small vascular neoplasm in the lateral aspect of the lower pole of the left kidney (**b**).

An elderly woman was referred for examination because of a right renal mass noted on intravenous urography at another hospital. At right nephrectomy, a renal cell carcinoma of the kidney was found. Chemotherapy was started for treatment of the left kidney lesion.

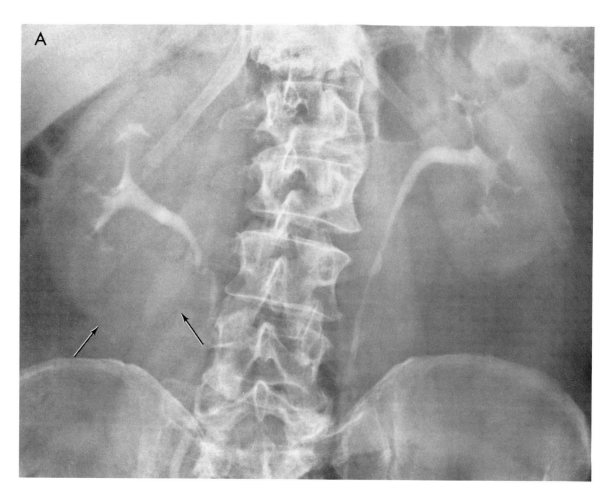

Comment: The importance of the flush aortogram in the study of renal mass lesions as a means of evaluating the opposite kidney is nicely demonstrated here. Had this procedure been omitted and only a right selective study performed, the unsuspected small neoplasm of the left kidney would have gone unrecognized.

Whether this case represents a primary carcinoma of the right kidney with a metastasis to the left kidney or two primary carcinomas really cannot be answered since histologically the two lesions might be identical. The former is thought to be more likely since metastasis from a renal carcinoma to the opposite kidney is not uncommon and was found in 11% of patients with renal adenocarcinoma in an autopsy series of 523 cases. On the other hand, bilateral carcinomas are considered extremely rare (less than 1%).*

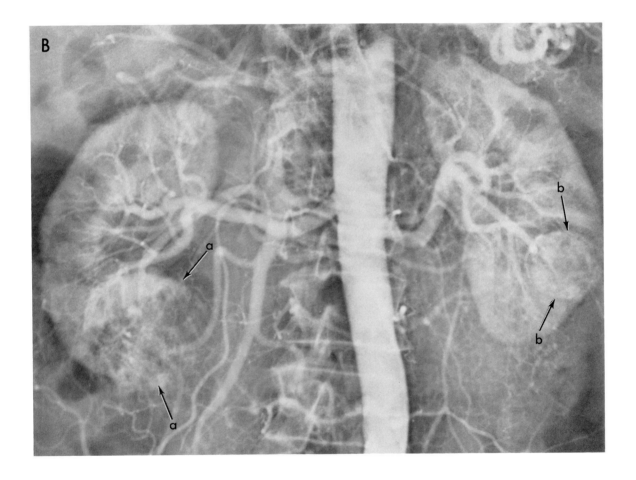

* Bennington, J. C., and Kradjian, R. M.: *Renal Carcinoma* (Philadelphia: W. B. Saunders Company, 1967).

Figure 46 · Bilateral Carcinoma / 147

Figure 47.—Renal cell carcinoma: incidental finding.

A, intravenous urogram, anteroposterior projection: Revealing obstruction of the left collecting system due to an opaque calculus at the ureterovesical junction (**a**). An unsuspected well-defined mass is seen in the midportion of the right kidney (**arrows**).

(*Continued* on p. 150.)

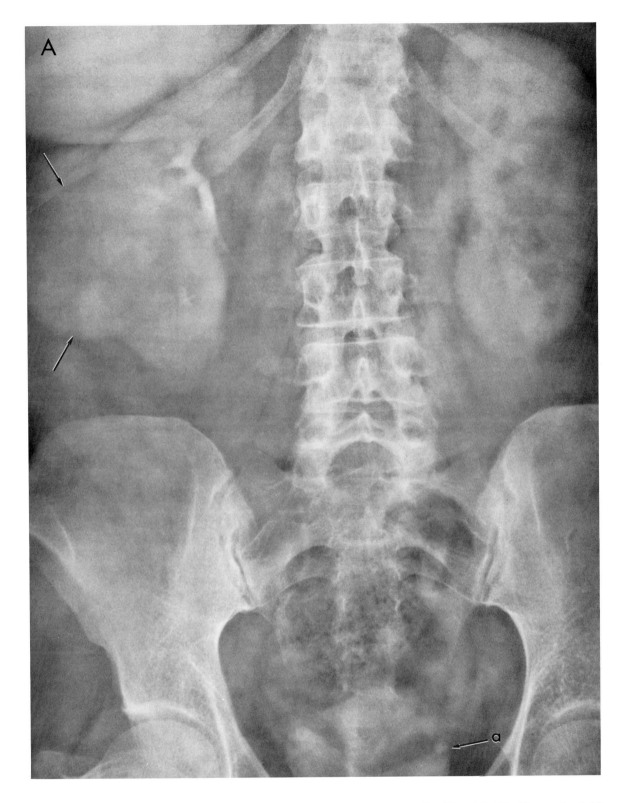

Figure 47 · Carcinoma as Incidental Finding / 149

Figure 47 (cont.).—Renal cell carcinoma: incidental finding.

B, right selective arteriogram, arterial phase, anteroposterior view: Demonstrating a number of neoplastic vessels coursing over the tumor at the lateral margin of the lower pole (**arrows**).

C, same study, nephrogram phase: Showing that most of the mass is cystic, with a thick wall. There are areas of tumor stain (**x**). The angiographic findings are those of a partially necrotic neoplasm.

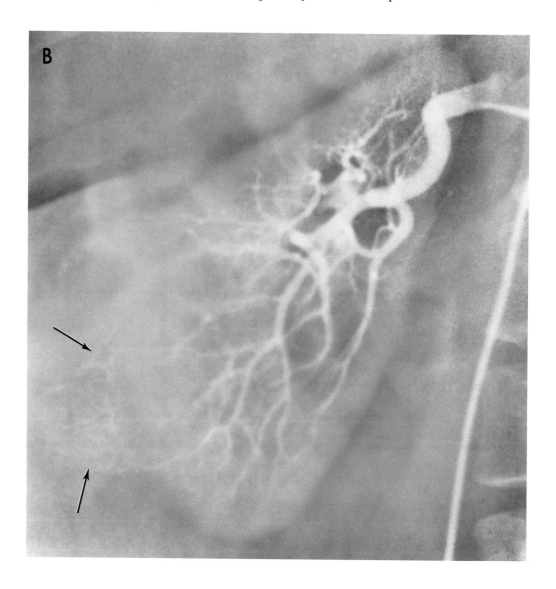

A woman of 43 was hospitalized because of left renal colic. She had no history of previous renal problems. Pathologic diagnosis of the surgical specimen was cystic clear cell carcinoma.

Comment: The right renal cell carcinoma was an incidental finding, brought to attention because of the left ureterovesical junction calculus. The prognosis for such a neoplasm is much better than for those that cause clinical symptoms.

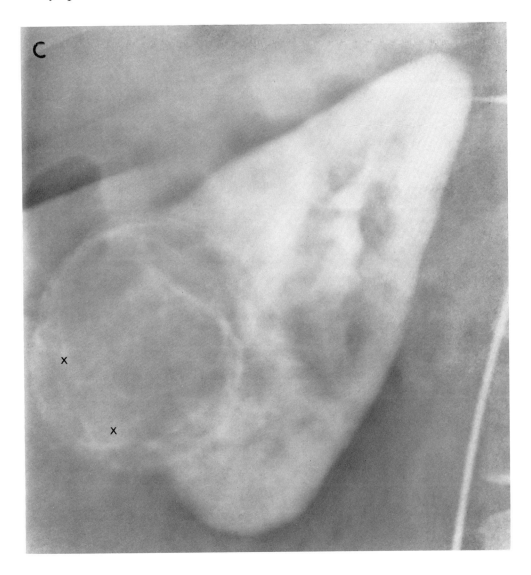

Figure 47 · Carcinoma as Incidental Finding / 151

Figure 48.—Renal cell carcinoma associated with a staghorn calculus.

A, intravenous urogram, anteroposterior projection: Revealing a staghorn calculus filling the left renal pelvis, infundibular and calyceal structures that produces a castlike appearance. A large mass occupies the lower pole of the kidney (**arrows**).

B, left renal arteriogram, anteroposterior view: Demonstrating at the

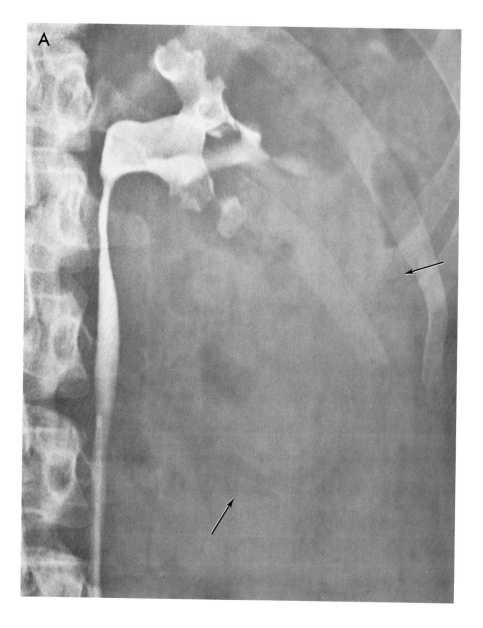

lower pole a moderately vascular tumor. Numerous small irregular tortuous vessels are seen throughout the mass, together with focal areas of contrast pooling or stasis that produce a blotchy type of tumor stain (**arrows**).

A 46-year-old woman with left flank pain was hospitalized for surgery for the staghorn calculus that was known to be present. The urogram, however, disclosed the associated renal mass. A left nephrectomy was performed; pathologic diagnosis was renal cell carcinoma.

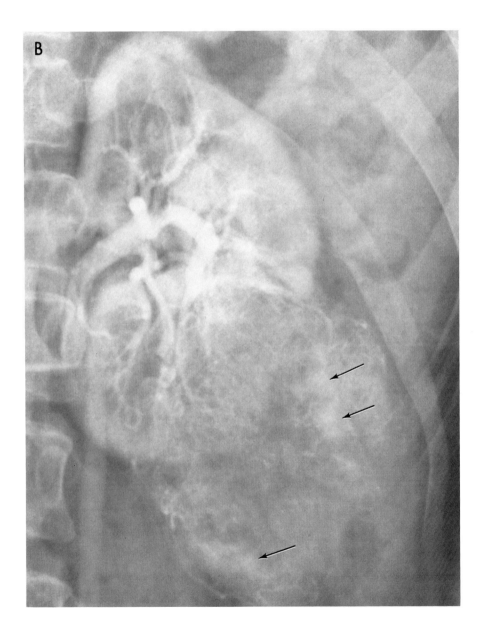

Figure 48 · Carcinoma with Staghorn Calculus / 153

Figure 49.—Carcinoma in a horseshoe kidney.

A, intravenous urogram, anteroposterior exposure: Demonstrating non-visualization of the collecting system on the left. Rotation of the right collecting system is characteristic of horseshoe kidney. A well-defined isthmus joins the lower pole of the kidneys (**arrows**). Curvilinear rimlike calcifications are present in the left kidney (**x**).

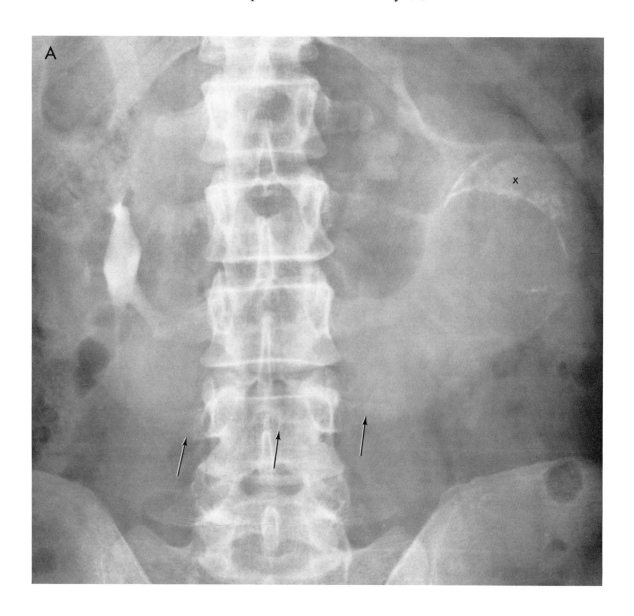

B, aortogram, late phase, anteroposterior view: Confirming the presence of a horseshoe kidney. There are two renal arteries to each kidney (**y**). The upper arteries are barely visible on this film, but the lower ones are well demonstrated. Note the nephrogram of the isthmus of the horseshoe kidney. Numerous tumor vessels are evident in the region of the calcification (**arrows**).

(*Continued* on p. 156.)

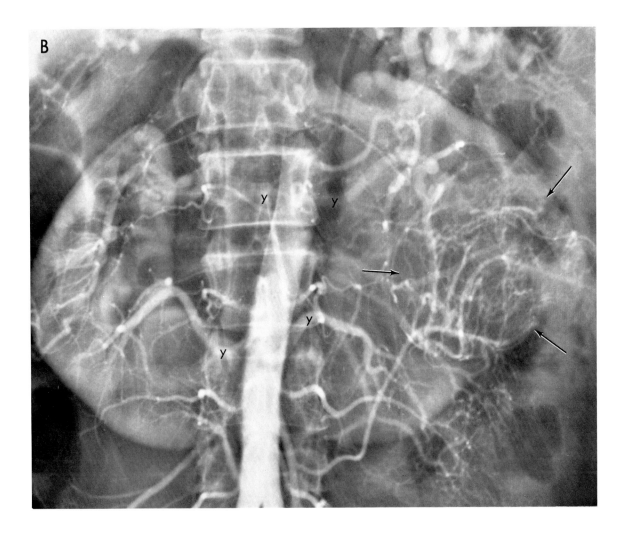

Figure 49 · Carcinoma in Horseshoe Kidney / 155

Figure 49 (cont.).—Carcinoma in a horseshoe kidney.

C, selective left renal arteriogram of the main (upper) renal artery, anteroposterior exposure: Demonstrating even more graphically than the aortogram (**B**) the abnormal vasculature. The vessels are irregularly dilated, distorted and disorganized. The pathologic vasculature is fairly well confined to the areas of calcification. The angiographic findings are typical of malignant tumor.

A man of 44, known to have horseshoe kidney, was hospitalized because of hematuria. At surgery the isthmus of the horseshoe kidney was split and a left nephrectomy performed. Pathologic diagnosis was renal cell carcinoma.

Comment: This combination of lesions, although rare, has been reported.* The arteriogram in this instance clearly established the suspected diagnosis and outlined the vascular anatomy. Angiography is indicated in cases of renal anomalies of all types, particularly if there is any suspicion of associated tumor.

Figure 49, courtesy of Dr. R. P. Cavallino, Summit, N.J.

---

* Shoup, G. D.; Pollack, H. W., and Dou, J. H.: Adenocarcinoma occurring in a horseshoe kidney: Report of a case and review of the literature, Arch. Surg. (Chicago) 84:413, 1962.

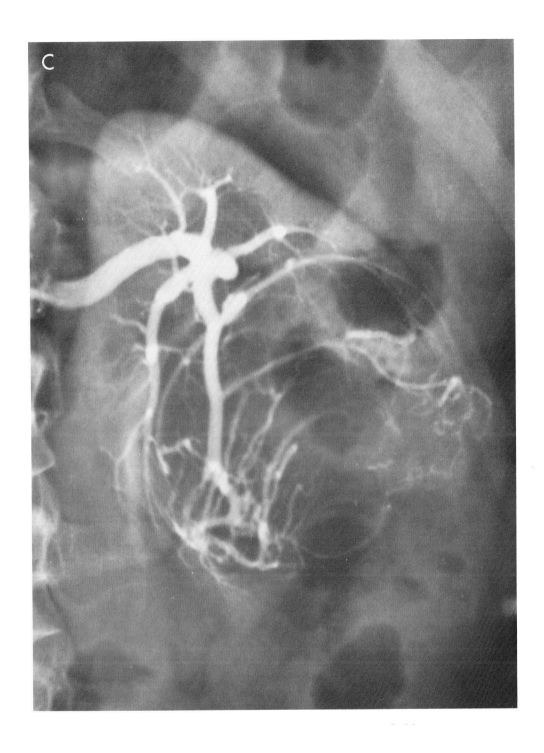

Figure 49 · Carcinoma in Horseshoe Kidney / 157

Figure 50.—Carcinoma in a kidney with duplicated collecting system.

A, intravenous urogram, anteroposterior view: Delineating a bifid pelvis on the left. On the right the collecting system in the upper pole of the kidney (**x**) is not demonstrated. The configuration suggests a duplicated collecting system.

B, right retrograde pyelogram, anteroposterior exposure: Confirming the presence of complete duplication of the right collecting system and demonstrating the upper portion. Note that there is no displacement or distortion of the calyx.

C, aortogram, anteroposterior view: Revealing a few clusters of abnormal vessels in the upper pole of the right kidney (**arrows**), indicating a malignant lesion in this area. The aorta and other vessels are normal.

A 44-year-old woman entered the hospital because of right flank pain and hematuria. Right nephrectomy was performed. A renal cell carcinoma was confined to the upper pole of the kidney.

Comment: The need for angiography in the study of difficult renal cases is well shown in this case. No distortion or displacement of collecting system structures was detected. But angiography was performed because blood was seen coming from the ureter draining the upper pole on cystoscopy. Also, a satisfactory explanation for nonvisualization of the upper collecting system on urography was not apparent. Angiography provided the diagnosis in this perplexing case.

Figure 50, courtesy of Bosniak, M. A.; Scheff, S., and Kaufman, S.: Localized hydronephrosis masquerading as a renal neoplasm, J. Urol. 99:241, 1968.

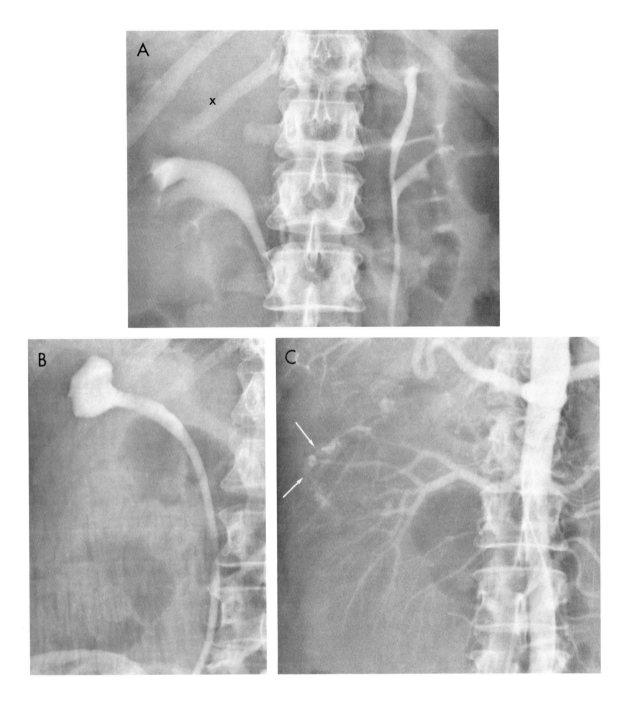

Figure 50 · Carcinoma with Renal Anomaly / 159

Figure 51.—Bilateral lesions—right renal cell carcinoma and left adrenal adenoma.

A, intravenous urogram, anteroposterior exposure: Revealing a large mass at the lower pole of the right kidney (**arrows**) and associated calyceal distortion. The upper pole of the left kidney is tilted laterally, with greater distance between the upper pole calyx and spine on the left than on the right. Two faceted gallstones overlie the right kidney (**a**).

B, aortogram, late phase, anteroposterior view: Demonstrating a large vascular neoplasm of the lower pole of the right kidney. Note also the vascular lesion at the upper pole of the left kidney (**x**).

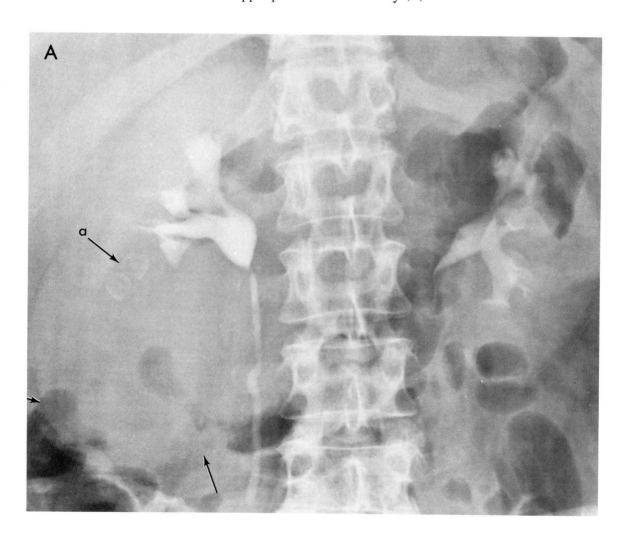

A woman of 55 entered the hospital for evaluation of a palpable right-sided mass. Right nephrectomy for a renal cell carcinoma was performed, as well as left adrenalectomy for a benign adenoma. The left kidney was normal.

Comment: The importance of flush aortography to help detect all lesions in the abdomen is well demonstrated. Presence of the left-sided lesion was not completely appreciated on the urogram but became clear on the aortogram, though its nature was not evident until surgery. From the angiogram it was not certain whether the vascular tumor on the left side was renal or adrenal and whether it represented a metastasis from the large right renal malignancy or was another primary neoplasm. Its benign nature was not suspected until surgery.

Figure 51, courtesy of Drs. S. S. Siegelman and S. Sprayregen, Montefiore Hospital, New York.

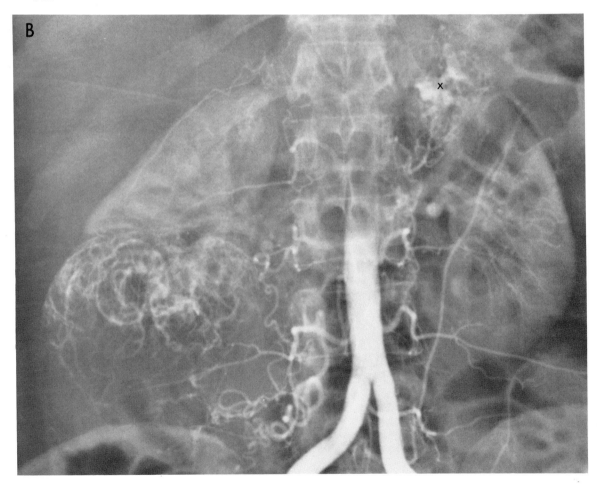

Figure 51 · Bilateral Renal and Adrenal Lesions / 161

Figure 52.—Renal cell carcinoma of the right kidney with shrunken pyelonephritic left kidney.

A, intravenous urogram, anteroposterior projection: Demonstrating nonvisualization of the collecting system and a large renal shadow on the right (**arrows**). A shrunken, pyelonephritic left kidney with diminished cortex and calyceal dilatation is present.

B, aortogram, anteroposterior view: Delineating tumor vesesls around the hilus of the right kidney and lower pole (**arrows**), indicating a malignant lesion. Two attenuated vessels supply the small left kidney; the intrarenal

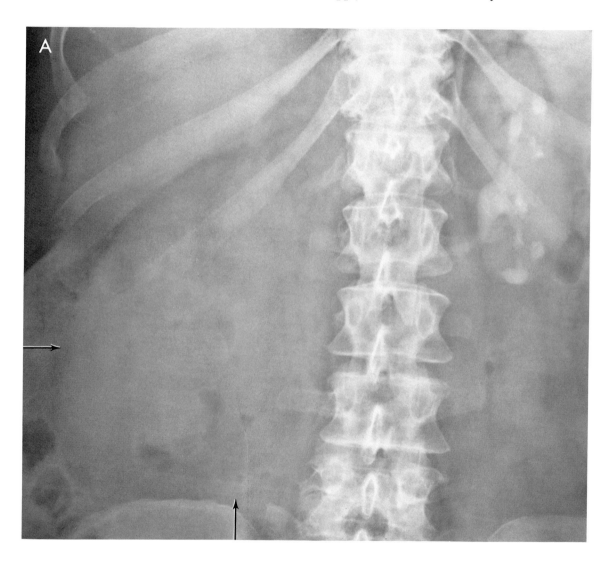

branches are diminished and truncated—an appearance consistent with the arterial pattern seen in chronic atrophic pyelonephritis.

A woman of 56 was hospitalized because of gross hematuria. Differential function studies indicated that the left kidney could sustain life and a right nephrectomy was performed. The lesion was a renal cell carcinoma. She did well for a year and then was lost to follow-up.

Comment: Evaluation of the blood supply to both kidneys is important, particularly if nephrectomy is contemplated.

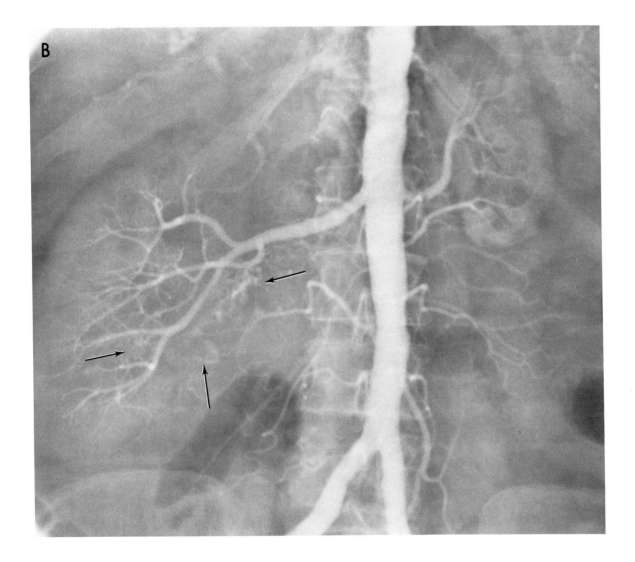

Figure 52 · Carcinoma: Opposite Kidney Pyelonephrotic / 163

Figure 53.—Small carcinoma fed only by an accessory renal artery.

A, nephrotomogram, anteroposterior projection: Delineating a lucency of 1 cm diameter in the cortex of the midpole of the right kidney (**x**). There is also an ill-defined, partly lucent area at the lower pole (**arrows**). Note that the margin of the renal contour of the lower pole is not well defined.

B, selective right renal arteriogram, *main renal artery*, arterial phase: Demonstrating that the vessels visualized are essentially normal. There is some stretching of vessels around a small cystic structure in the cortex in the midportion of the kidney. Note some overflow filling of an accessory renal artery to the lower pole (**arrow**). No abnormal vascularity is seen.

C, same study, nephrogram phase: Confirming the presence of a small cyst in the cortex (**x**). There is no nephrogram in the lower pole of the kidney, indicating that an accessory artery is supplying it.

(*Continued* on p. 166.)

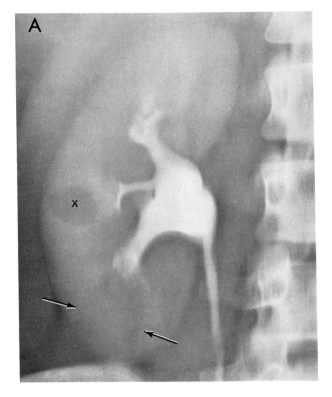

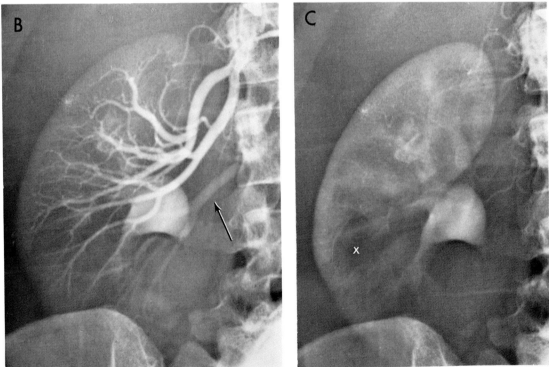

Figure 53 · Carcinoma with Unusual Blood Supply / 165

Figure 53 (cont.).—Small carcinoma fed only by an accessory renal artery.

D, selective *accessory* right renal arteriogram, arterial phase: Clearly demonstrating a small collection of tumor vessels in the lower pole (**arrow**). The vascular supply to the tumor comes only from the accessory artery.

E, same study, nephrogram phase: Clearly visualizing the lower portion of the kidney. Stasis of contrast medium in the tumor vessels precisely delineates the size of the small neoplasm (**arrow**).

A woman of 42 was studied radiologically after a nodule was palpated in the right kidney during hysterectomy. An intravenous urogram revealed an ill-defined mass at the lower pole. At right nephrectomy a renal cell carcinoma 2.5 cm in diameter was found.

Comment: The small carcinoma was fed solely by a small accessory vessel. This unusual angiographic series confirms the need to perform midstream aortography plus selective arteriography in the investigation of renal masses. Aortography clearly outlines the anatomy and will not allow an accessory vessel to escape detection. At the same time, absence of some portion of the nephrogram following a selective arteriogram (**C**) should alert the radiologist to the possible presence of an accessory vessel.

Figure 53, courtesy of Dr. L. R. Barris, Newark, N.J., and Siegelman, S. S., *et al.:* Incomplete renal angiography: The naked calyx sign, J. Urol. 103:27, 1970.

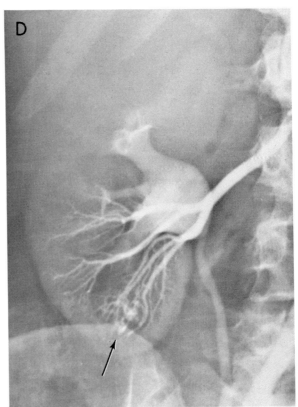

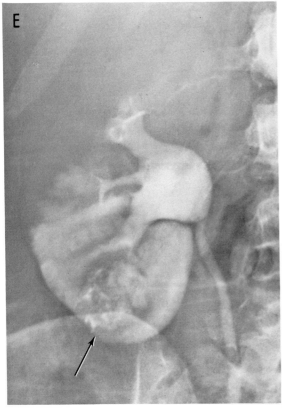

Figure 53 · Carcinoma with Unusual Blood Supply / 167

Figure 54.—Huge capsular artery originating directly from the aorta and supplying a large renal carcinoma.

A, aortogram, early phase, anteroposterior exposure: Delineating a large vascular neoplasm of the right kidney with typical neoplastic vessels (**arrows**). Note also the large capsular artery (**a**) arising from the aorta just below the main renal artery and extending inferiorly around the lowermost margin of the mass.

B, same study, later phase: Defining the capsular artery supplying the lower margin of the neoplasm as it courses upward along the lateral margin of the tumor (**a**). In the main portion of the tumor there are typical abnormal vessels with pooling of contrast medium and venous aneurysm formation (**x**).

A man of 63 was studied because of a large right-sided abdominal mass. An intravenous urogram revealed a mass at the lower pole of the right kidney. Nephrectomy by right thoracoabdominal approach was performed and a renal cell carcinoma removed.

Comment: The unusual vessel supplying a large part of the tumor probably represents an enlarged capsular artery. Hypertrophy of capsular arteries feeding vascular renal neoplasms is not uncommon (see Fig. 32). However, these vessels are usually early branches of the main renal artery. Occasionally these vessels arise from the aorta separately but are not often seen because of their small size. In this case the vessel hypertrophied to feed the renal carcinoma. The vessel probably would have been missed had flush aortography not been performed. Aware of its existence, the surgeon was able to identify and tie it during nephrectomy. The radiographic delineation of the entire renal vascular supply prior to surgery has contributed significantly to the reduction of complications at the time of nephrectomy (see Freed *et al.* below).

Figure 54, courtesy of Freed, S. Z.; Caplan, L. H., and Bosniak, M. A.: The role of renal arteriography in the management of renal carcinoma, Surg., Gynec. & Obst. 123:1303, 1966.

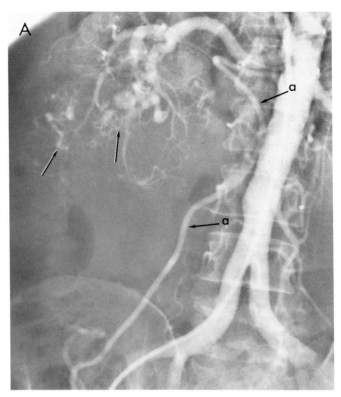

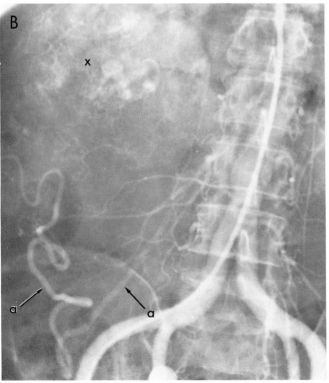

Figure 54 · Carcinoma with Unusual Blood Supply / 169

Figure 55.—Huge spermatic artery feeding a renal cell carcinoma.

A, selective right renal arteriogram, anteroposterior view: Revealing a large vascular malignant lesion occupying the lower portion of the kidney.

B, selective right spermatic arteriogram: Delineating a hypertrophied spermatic artery (**arrow**) that gives off numerous branches which contribute to the vascular supply of the neoplasm.

A 51-year-old man was studied because of a right renal mass. Intravenous urography revealed a huge mass at the lower pole of the right kidney.

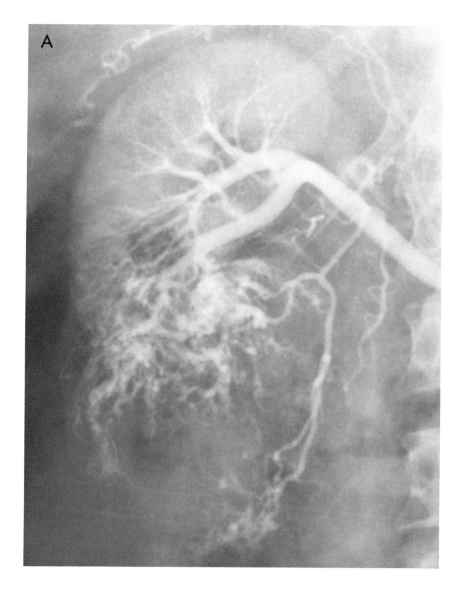

During nephrectomy for removal of a renal cell carcinoma the spermatic artery was identified and ligated.

Comment: Hypertrophy of spermatic arteries feeding vascular renal neoplasms is quite rare. Another instance of a spermatic artery feeding a retroperitoneal neoplasm is depicted in Figure 72, *B*. The spermatic artery gives off some small branches to the ureter and the retroperitoneal space as it courses inferiorly. In this case it hypertrophied to help supply the retroperitoneal extension of the neoplasm. Knowledge of its presence is important to the surgeon for safe performance of nephrectomy.

Figure 55, courtesy of Dr. Ervin Philipps, Woodland, Calif.

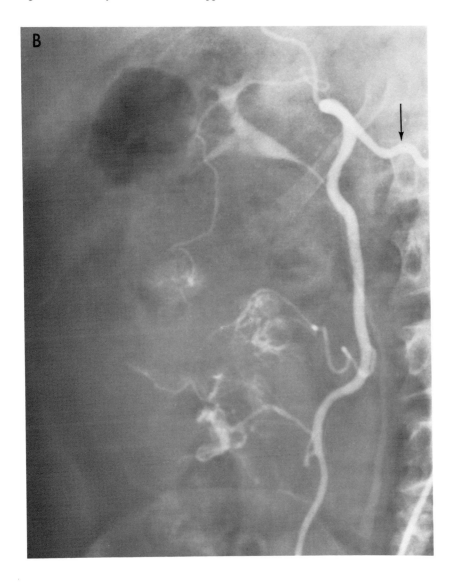

Figure 55 · Carcinoma with Unusual Blood Supply / 171

Figure 56.—Extension of renal carcinoma outside the capsule, with supply by a lumbar artery.

A, selective right renal arteriogram, anteroposterior exposure: Showing the entire kidney filled with tumor vessels. Note, however, that the large mass extends laterally from the kidney (**x**) and is not supplied by renal vessels. On the preliminary aortogram this area was seen to be supplied by a lumbar artery.

(*Continued* on p. 174.)

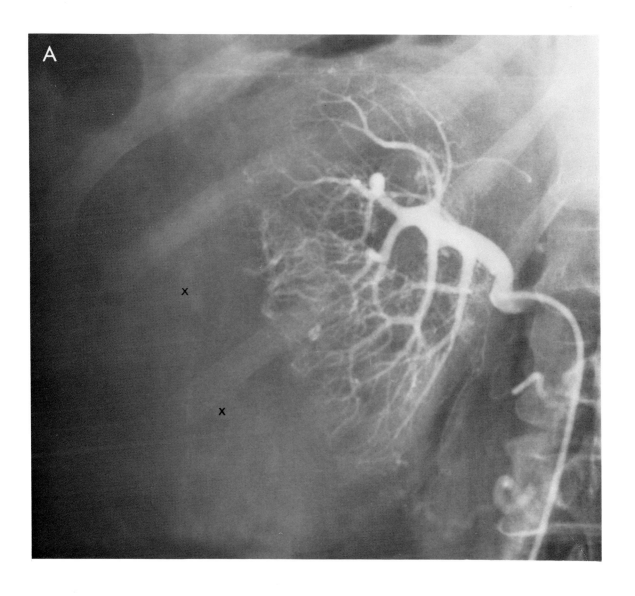

Figure 56 · Carcinoma with Unusual Blood Supply / 173

Figure 56 (cont.).—Extension of renal carcinoma outside the capsule, with supply by a lumbar artery.

B, selective lumbar (L3) arteriogram, early phase: Disclosing the hypertrophied vessel which passes upward to supply the outer portion of the large renal tumor that extends outside the capsule into the perirenal space (**arrows**).

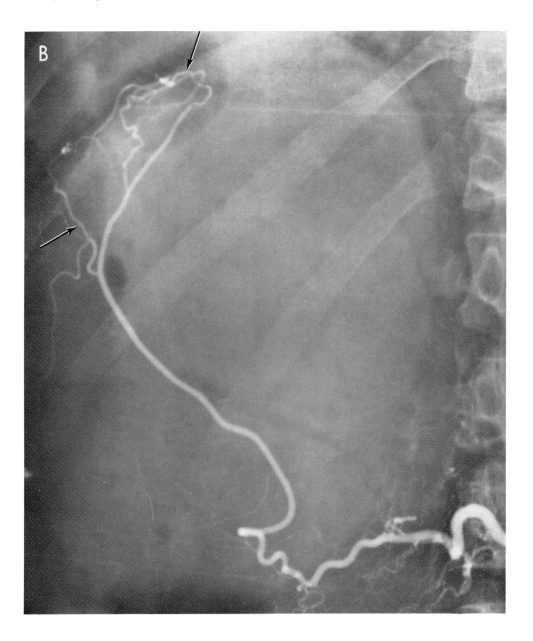

C, same study, late phase: Delineating tumor vessels and stain extending into the perirenal tissues (**arrows**).

Comment: The extent of renal carcinoma into the perirenal tissues can be evaluated by angiography. Supply of the tumor by lumbar arteries indicates that the neoplasm has extended beyond the renal capsule into the surrounding tissues.

Figure 56, courtesy of Dr. Ervin Philipps, Woodland, Calif.

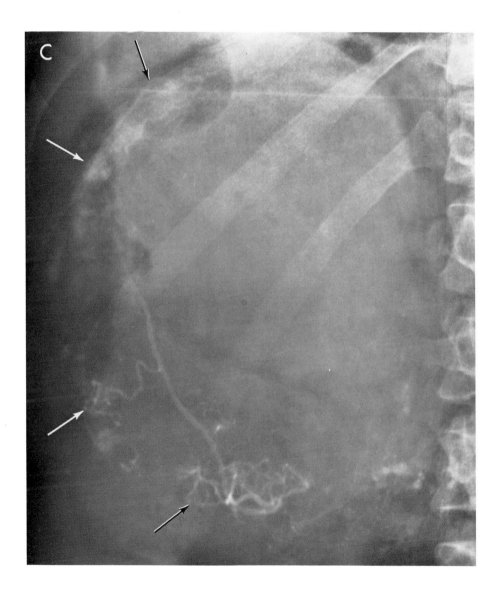

Figure 56 · Carcinoma with Unusual Blood Supply / 175

Figure 57.—Renal cell carcinoma with huge arteriovenous fistula.

A, intravenous urogram, anteroposterior exposure: Showing a mass at the lower pole of the left kidney with splaying of the lower and middle pole calyces. There is notching of the incompletely filled upper ureter.

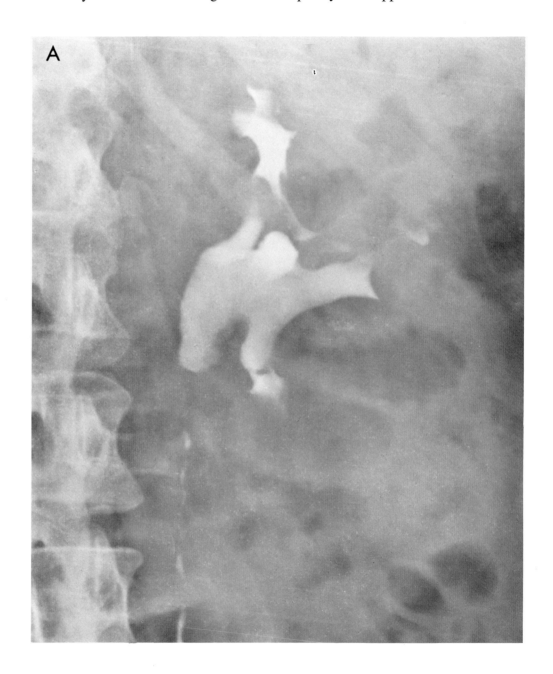

B, aortogram, early film, anteroposterior view: Delineating three large renal arteries supplying the left kidney. A large vascular tumor involves the middle and lower poles.

(*Continued* on p. 178.)

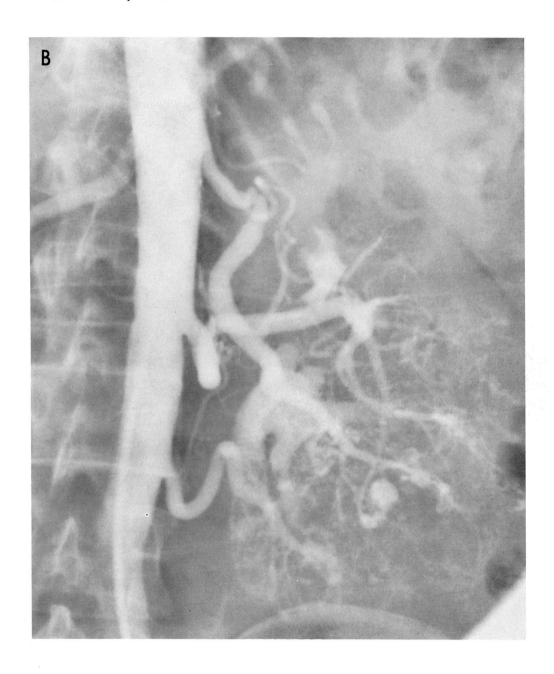

Figure 57 · Carcinoma with Arteriovenous Fistula / 177

Figure 57 (cont.).—Renal cell carcinoma with huge arteriovenous fistula.

C, aortogram 1 second after **B**: Revealing early opacification of the left renal vein (**y**) and inferior vena cava (**x**) while the contrast agent is still in the lower aorta and iliac arteries. The defect in the renal vein (**a**) represents tumor extension.

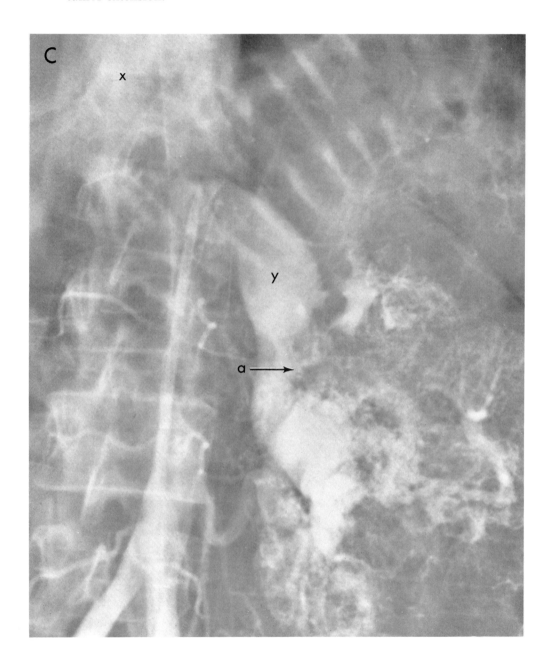

D, aortogram 0.75 second after **C:** Delineating a hypertrophied ureteral artery (**b**) that contributes to the vascular supply of the neoplasm. There is early opacification of the ovarian vein (**c**). Note further opacification of the inferior vena cava (**x**).

(*Continued* on p. 180.)

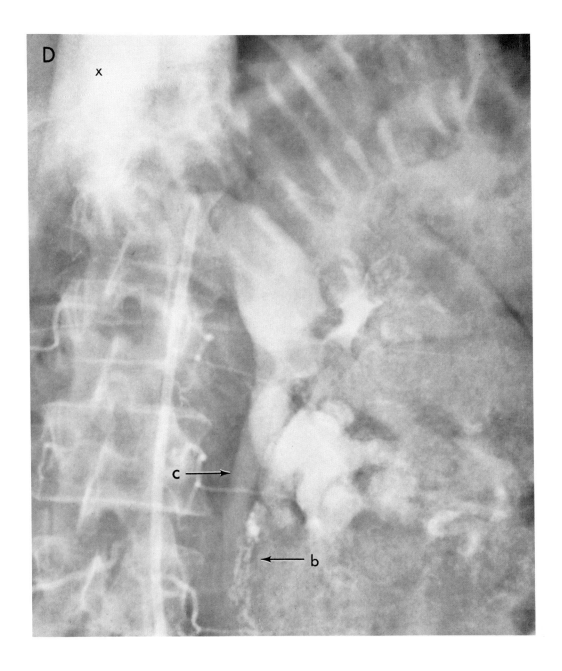

Figure 57 · Carcinoma with Arteriovenous Fistula / 179

Figure 57 (cont.).—Renal cell carcinoma with huge arteriovenous fistula.

E, aortogram 0.75 second after **D**: Showing further retrograde filling of the large dilated ovarian vein (**c**).

F, surgical specimen: Showing replacement of the middle and lower poles of the kidney by renal cell carcinoma. The renal vein was invaded by tumor.

A 40-year-old woman was hospitalized because of hypertension.

Comment: Kidney carcinoma is frequently vascular and composed of numerous small arteriovenous fistulas and shunts. Early venous filling is therefore not uncommon with renal malignancies. Occasionally, however, as in this case, the degree of arteriovenous shunting may lead to a massive arteriovenous fistula which can be confused arteriographically and hemodynamically with arteriovenous fistulas due to other causes (see Bosniak below).

Arteriovenous fistulas occurring anywhere in the body will lead to systolic hypertension with a low diastolic pressure and a wide pulse pressure. When an arteriovenous fistula occurs in the kidney, however, diastolic as well as systolic hypertension will usually result. This is presumably due to associated renal ischemia. Arteriovenous fistulas can lead to serious hemodynamic changes including high output congestive heart failure (see Fig. 58).

The notching of the ureter in this case was caused by the ureteral artery which hypertrophied due to increased blood flow to this highly vascular lesion.

Figure 57, courtesy of Bosniak, M. A.: Radiographic manifestations of massive arteriovenous fistula in renal carcinoma, Radiology 85:454, 1965.

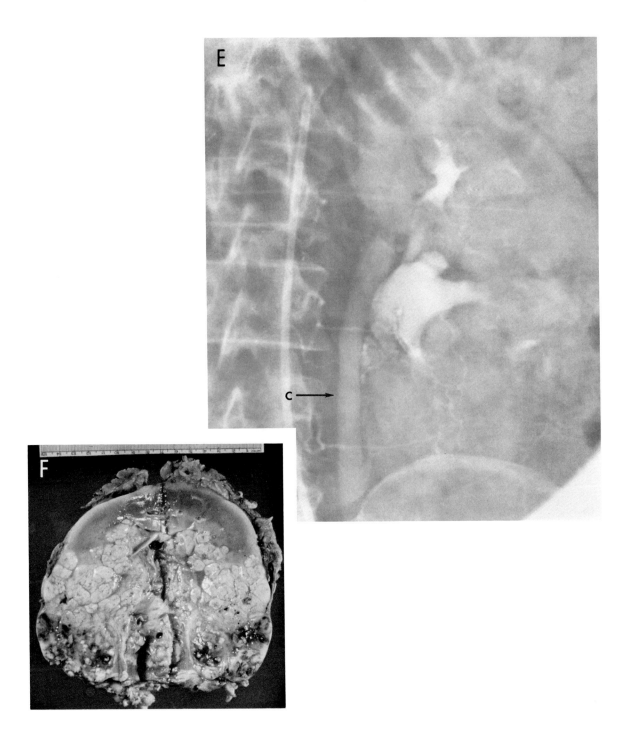

Figure 57 · Carcinoma with Arteriovenous Fistula / 181

Figure 58.—Renal cell carcinoma with massive arteriovenous fistula.

A, aortogram, early phase, anteroposterior projection: Showing a hypertrophied right renal artery (**arrow**) supplying a large vascular tumor of the right kidney. Early filling of the inferior vena cava (**x**) indicates an extensive arteriovenous fistula.

B, same study 0.5 second later: Revealing the extent of the arteriovenous shunting. The inferior vena cava (**x**) is now well opacified while contrast medium is still in the distal aorta.

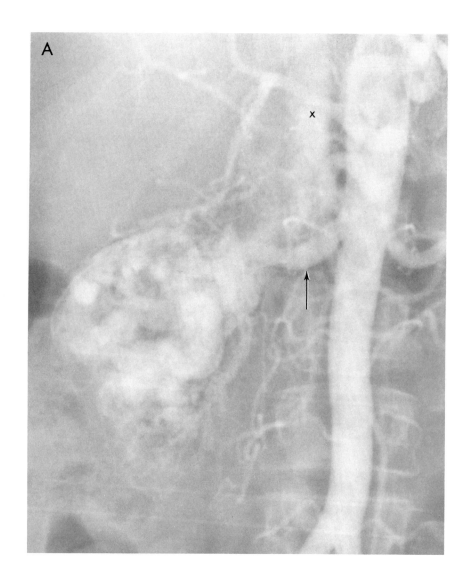

On hospitalization this woman of 61 had a blood pressure reading of 240/120 mm. Hg. A preoperative dye dilution study of cardiac output indicated an increased rate (4.1 liters/min/m²). A right nephrectomy was performed and a renal cell carcinoma removed. Postoperative blood pressure was 140/80 mm Hg and remained at this level for at least a year. A follow-up cardiac output study revealed that the cardiac index had returned to normal limits (3.26 liters/min/m²) (see Wise *et al.* below).

Figure 58, courtesy of Wise, G. W.; Bosniak, M. A., and Hudson, P. B.: Arteriovenous fistula associated with renal cell carcinoma of the kidney, Brit. J. Urol. 39:170, 1967.

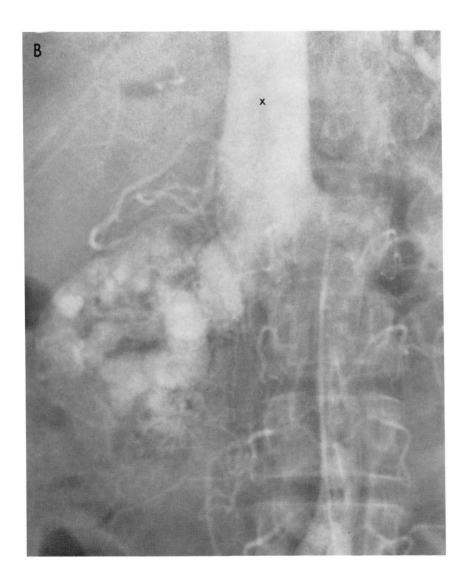

Figure 58 · Carcinoma with Arteriovenous Fistula / 183

Figure 59.—Carcinoma and cyst in the same kidney.

A, selective right renal arteriogram, arterial phase, anteroposterior projection: Revealing two lesions of the right kidney. The one along the upper lateral margin is avascular with displacement of vessels (**a**). That at the lower pole is hypovascular, but vessels of abnormal appearance are seen at its base and an enlarged capsular artery supplies the wall of the lesion (**b**). Some irregular calcification is also present in its wall (**c**).

B, same study, nephrogram phase: Showing a completely lucent upper lesion with thin wall and two spurs (**arrows**), indicating a simple benign cyst. The lower pole lesion contains areas of density (**x**) that represent pooling of contrast medium in the tumor tissue. A thick plaque of calcium forms part of the wall of the mass (**c**).

A man of 73 was referred because of frequency, urgency and nocturia. An intravenous urogram demonstrated a partially calcified mass over the lower pole of the right kidney. Right nephrectomy disclosed a large necrotic carcinoma of the lower pole and a simple cyst at the upper pole.

Comment: The incidence of carcinoma and cyst in the same kidney is put at 1–2%. In a study of 1007 consecutive cases of surgically proved renal cysts or tumors Emmett and his associates* at Mayo Clinic found 10 such cases. In eight the lesions were widely separated in the kidney, as in this case. Each lesion is well delineated angiographically, so correct diagnosis of cyst and tumor in the same kidney should pose no problems.

---

* Emmett, J. L.; Levine, S. R., and Woolner, L. B.: Co-existence of renal cyst and tumor, Brit. J. Urol. 35:403, 1963.

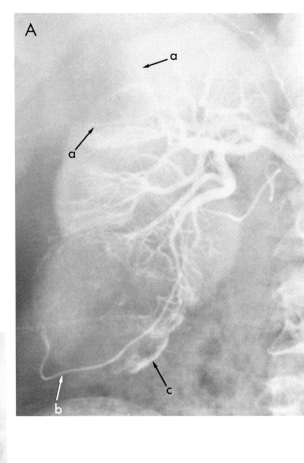

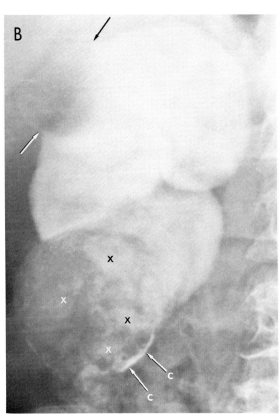

Figure 59 · Carcinoma and Cyst in Same Kidney / 185

Figure 60.—Tumor in the wall of a simple benign renal cyst.

A, selective left renal arteriogram, arterial phase, anteroposterior projection: Demonstrating normal intrarenal vascularity, and a large avascular mass projecting off the lower pole of the kidney which represents a benign

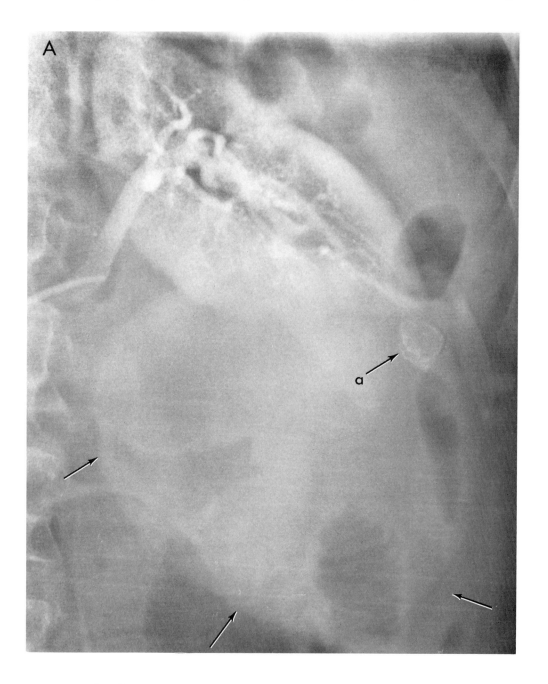

cyst (**arrows**). Note, however, the vessels to a small 2.0 cm nodule in the cyst wall (**a**).

B, same study, nephrogram phase: Delineating a small tumor nodule (**a**) in the wall of the large cyst.

(*Continued* on p. 188.)

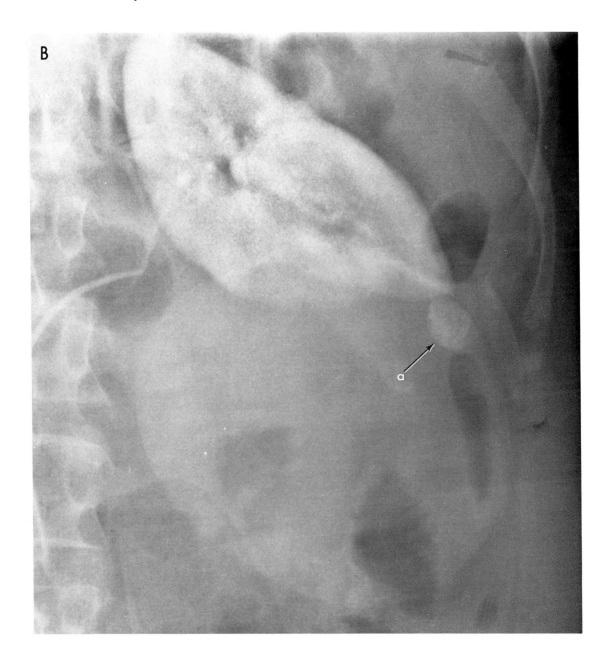

B

Figure 60 · Renal Tumor in Cyst Wall / 187

Figure 60 (cont.).—Tumor in the wall of a simple, benign renal cyst.

C, anteroposterior exposure following cyst puncture and instillation of iodine contrast agent and air, patient supine: Confirming the presence of a smooth-contoured cyst at the lower pole. A small nodule causes a negative filling defect (**a**) in the margin of the opaque cyst.

D, same study, with patient in right lateral decubitus position: Showing the air-fluid level in the cyst. The defect in air contrast (**a**) is due to the tumor nodule projecting into the cyst lumen.

A man of 43 was investigated because of a mass detected on barium enema study. Intravenous urography revealed a large mass at the lower pole of the left kidney. Exploratory surgery disclosed a 2 cm tumor in a large benign cyst. Biopsy revealed adenoma, and since the lesion measured less than 3 cm it was considered benign. A wedge resection of the neoplasm was performed, as well as unroofing of the cyst. Three years later the patient was well.

Comment: Whether one can detect a small neoplasm in the wall of an otherwise benign cyst is a constantly recurring question. Such an occasion is rare; this case and one other are the only examples we have found in an experience with several thousand nephrotomograms and arteriograms. None was found in the 1007 cases studied by the Mayo Clinic group. This case demonstrates that when this rare situation does occur it can be diagnosed by nephrotomography and angiography.

Figure 60, courtesy of Silverman, J. F., and Kilhenny, C: Tumor in the wall of a simple renal cyst: Report of a case, Radiology 93:95, 1969.

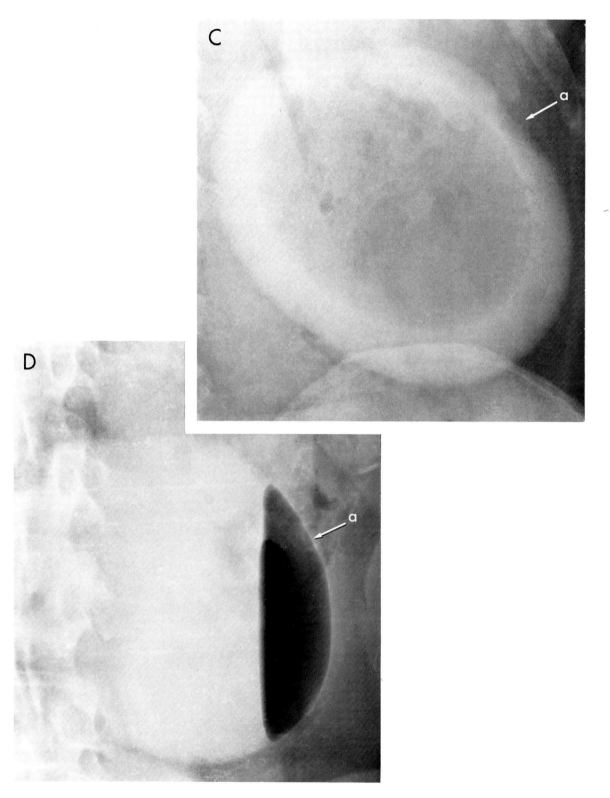

Figure 60 · Renal Tumor in Cyst Wall / 189

Figure 61.—Carcinoma in a polycystic kidney.

A, nephrotomogram, anteroposterior view: Showing the left kidney containing numerous cysts of various sizes and with distortion of the collecting system. The right kidney also shows calyceal distortion but few clearly defined cysts.

B, aortogram, anteroposterior projection: Delineating a large vascular neoplasm involving the right kidney and primarily fed by a hypertrophied renal artery branch (**a**). Many large neoplastic vessels are evident (**arrows**). The left kidney shows typical changes of cystic disease, with thin attenuated vessels displaced around the numerous cysts.

A man of 54 was hospitalized because of hypertension. An intravenous urogram revealed polycystic kidney disease, and nephrotomography and arteriography were advised for further evaluation. He refused to have surgery at the time of these studies but returned two years later because of hematuria and right flank pain. On right nephrectomy a renal cell carcinoma was found in a polycystic kidney.

Comment: Over 17 cases of malignant tumors in polycystic kidneys have been reported. Most authors believe that this is a chance occurrence and there is no relationship between these conditions. Most cases were not diagnosed preoperatively, being found at surgery or autopsy.* Routine radiologic studies do not detect a malignancy in a polycystic kidney. Angiography is necessary to make this diagnosis and should be performed in all cases of polycystic kidney disease in which there is hematuria or when there is radiologic evidence of calcification, calyceal amputation or significant difference in kidney size.

---

* Howard, R. M., and Young, J. D.: Two malignant tumors in a polycystic kidney, J. Urol. 102:162, 1969.

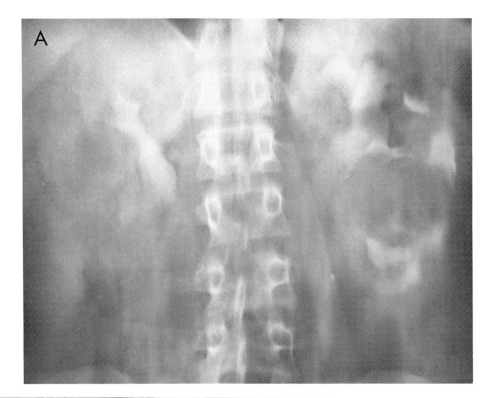

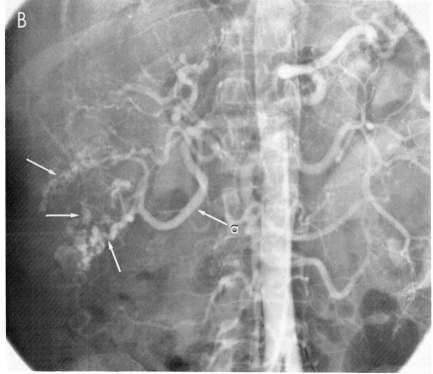

Figure 61 · Carcinoma in Polycystic Kidney / 191

Figure 62.—Tumor thrombus in inferior vena cava extending from a right renal carcinoma.

Inferior venacavogram, slight right posterior oblique projection: Showing a large tumor thrombus (**x**) filling the upper portion of the inferior vena cava. The cava, however, is not obstructed.

A man of 66 had gross hematuria. On intravenous urography the collecting system of the right kidney was not visualized. Renal angiography revealed a vascular carcinoma of the right kidney. At surgery a huge hypernephroma with tumor thrombus filling the renal vein and vena cava was partially resected.

Comment: Extension of renal carcinoma into the renal vein is relatively common. One-third to one-half of all renal adenocarcinomas show macroscopic involvement of the renal vein (surgical specimens). Prognosis is roughly one-half as good as when extension into the renal vein is not seen. Renal adenocarcinoma often extends directly into the venous structures and the inferior vena cava is involved in about 5% of cases.* The tumor sometimes extends up the cava to the right atrium. There are reports of sudden death due to massive pulmonary embolus by tumor thrombus following nephrectomy and manipulation of the cava.

Because of possible caval involvement, inferior venacavography should be used to search for extension of carcinoma into the cava. This and Figures 63–66 clearly outline the extensions of tumor into the cava—information important to the surgeon in planning and performing nephrectomy and in evaluating prognosis. All patients with renal carcinoma should have a cavogram if the kidney is not visualized on the urogram or findings on the angiogram suggest renal vein involvement, such as nonvisualization of the renal vein with drainage by collateral veins (Fig. 68) or the "striate pattern" (Fig. 65). Also, since upper and middle pole right renal carcinomas involve the cava twice as often as carcinomas in other portions of the kidney (probably due to the short right renal vein), patients with these lesions should be studied routinely by inferior venacavography.

---

* Riches, E.: *Tumors of the Kidney and Ureter* (Baltimore: Williams & Wilkins Company, 1964); McDonald, J. R., and Priestly, J. T.: Malignant tumors of the kidney: Surgical and prognostic significance of tumor thrombosis of the renal veins, Surg., Gynec. & Obst. 77: 295, 1943.

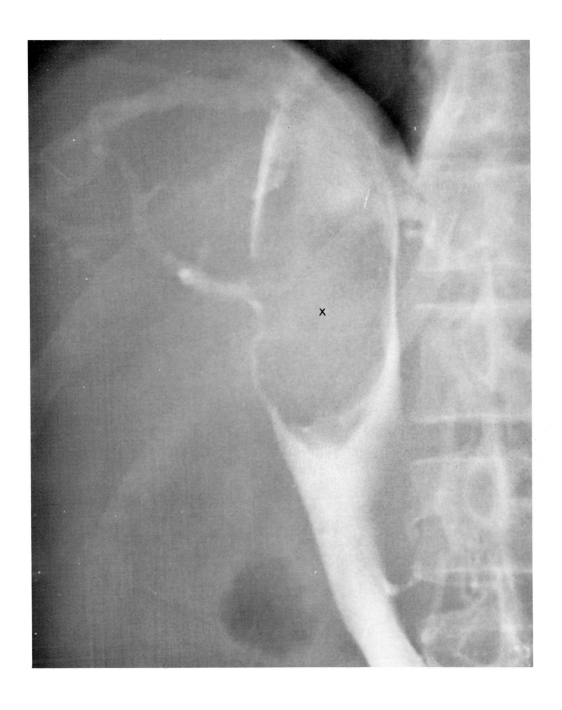

Figure 62 · Tumor Thrombus in Vena Cava / 193

Figure 63.—Extension of renal carcinoma into the inferior vena cava.

Inferior venacavogram, right posterior oblique projection: Showing the inferior vena cava to be invaded and obstructed (**x**) by extension from a large right renal carcinoma. Note collateral circulation through lumbar veins and azygos system (**a**) on the right and via the ascending lumbar vein (**b**) and hemiazygos system of veins on the left.

A man of 60 had a right upper quadrant mass. Intravenous urography failed to visualize the right renal collecting system. A renal angiogram revealed a large vascular neoplasm of the right kidney. Exploration disclosed an inoperable, large right renal cell carcinoma invading the wall and lumen of the inferior vena cava.

Figure 63, courtesy of Ferris, E. J.; Bosniak, M. A., and O'Connor, J. F.: An angiographic sign demonstrating extension of renal carcinoma into the renal vein and vena cava, Radiology 102:384, 1968.

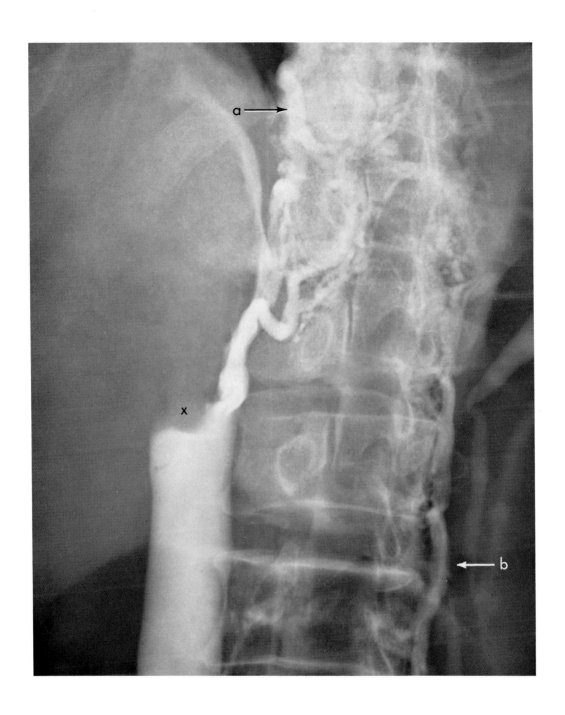

Figure 63 · Tumor Extension into Vena Cava / 195

Figure 64.—Extension of left renal cell carcinoma into the vena cava.

Inferior venacavogram, slight right posterior oblique projection: Showing a large tumor thrombus involving the inferior vena cava (**a**) as a direct extension of a left renal carcinoma. Some reflux of contrast medium into the right renal vein (**b**) has occurred. Collateral circulation through lumbar veins and the azygos system drains the cava.

A 48-year-old woman was hospitalized because of hematuria. An intravenous urogram revealed a mass at the lower pole of the left kidney, and a renal angiogram demonstrated a vascular neoplasm of the left kidney.

Figure 64, courtesy of Ferris, E. J.; Bosniak, M. A., and O'Connor, J. F.: An angiographic sign demonstrating extension of renal carcinoma into the renal vein and vena cava, Radiology 102:384, 1968.

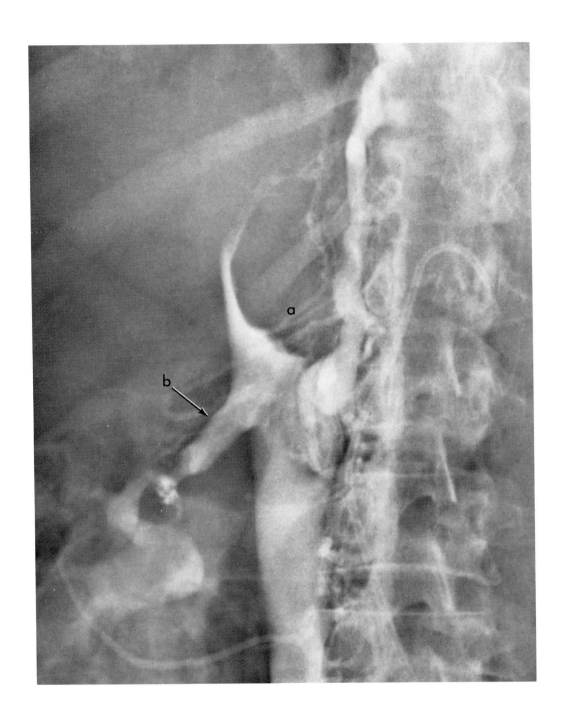

Figure 64 · Tumor Extension into Vena Cava / 197

Figure 65.—Extension of renal carcinoma into the inferior vena cava.

A, selective right renal arteriogram, late arterial phase, anteroposterior projection: Demonstrating a large vascular carcinoma with abnormal vascularity throughout the entire kidney. Note numerous streaming vessels (**arrows**) arising from the superior margin of the kidney and extending cephalad. These vessels are feeding the carcinoma which has extended into the renal vein and inferior vena cava (see **B**).

B, inferior venacavogram, anteroposterior exposure: Showing a large tumor thrombus (**x**) which occupies the inferior vena cava and extends into the right atrium.

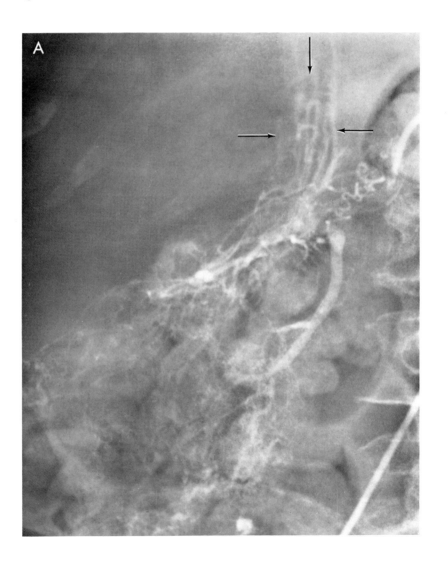

A woman of 70 was hospitalized because of hematuria and a right-sided abdominal mass. Intravenous urography revealed a mass involving the lower pole of the right kidney.

Comment: This "striate" appearance of vessels visualized in the angiogram is best seen when epinephrine angiography is used and is quite characteristic and diagnostic of extension of tumor from the kidney into the renal vein and cava.

Figure 65, courtesy of Ferris, E. J.; Bosniak, M. A., and O'Connor, J. F.: An angiographic sign demonstrating extension of renal carcinoma into the renal vein and vena cava, Radiology 102:384, 1968.

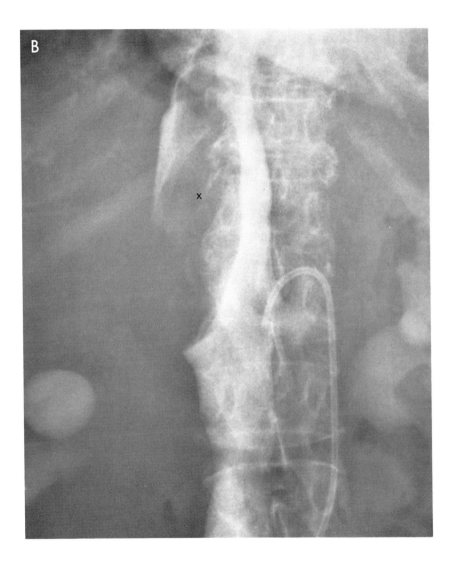

Figure 65 · Tumor Extension into Vena Cava / 199

Figure 66.—Obstruction of the inferior vena cava by extension of a renal cell carcinoma.

Inferior venacavogram, anteroposterior projection: Showing complete occlusion of the inferior vena cava (**x**). Collateral circulation is through the lumbar and vertebral plexus of veins to the azygos system.

A 46-year-old man was hospitalized because of weakness and leg edema. Intravenous urography revealed a mass distorting the calyces of a poorly functioning right kidney. Renal angiography disclosed a huge vascular carcinoma (see Fig. 70). Surgical exploration confirmed the radiographic findings.

Figure 66, courtesy of Ferris, E. J.; Bosniak, M. A., and O'Connor, J. F.: An angiographic sign demonstrating extension of renal carcinoma into the renal vein and vena cava, Radiology 102:384, 1968.

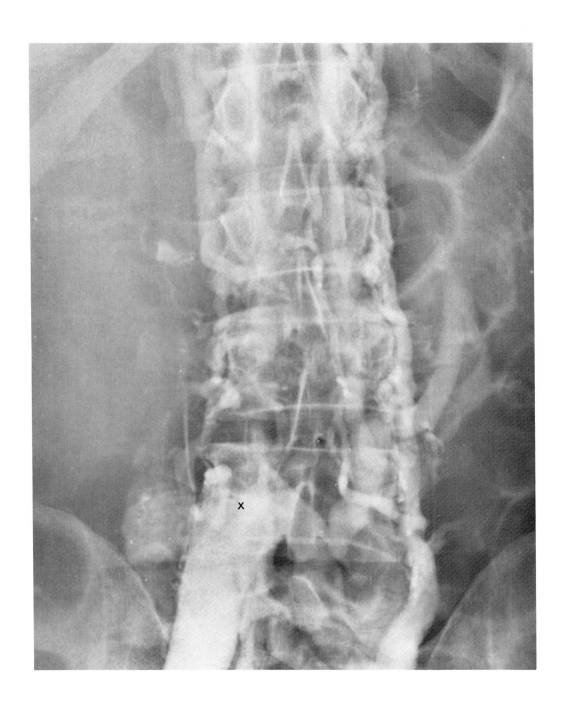

Figure 66 · Tumor Extension into Vena Cava / 201

Figure 67.—Renal venography in carcinoma of the kidney.

A, aortogram, anteroposterior projection: Delineating abundant tumor vessels at the upper pole and hilus of the left kidney (**arrows**).

B, selective left renal venogram, anteroposterior exposure: Clearly demonstrating the left renal vein and its tributaries. The sharp cutoff of the main renal vein (**a**) is caused by tumor invasion. Retrograde filling of collateral venous pathways is evident from the enlarged adrenal vein superiorly (**b**), the spermatic vein inferiorly (**c**) and a large capsular vein draining into the spermatic vein.

A 75-year-old man entered the hospital because of vague abdominal pain. Intravenous urography revealed bilateral renal masses. (The right renal lesion proved to be a benign cyst.) A left nephrectomy was performed. Pathologic diagnosis was renal cell carcinoma.

Comment: Selective renal phlebography is an adjunctive angiographic technique for estimating the full extent of a renal cell carcinoma. It has both prognostic and therapeutic application. Since venous invasion is so common in renal malignancy, its absence in a large lesion (whose arteriographic pattern is not typical for renal carcinoma) might suggest that the lesion is a benign tumor or an inflammatory process (see Kahn below).

Figure 67, courtesy of Kahn, P. C.: Selective venography in renal parenchymal disease, Radiology 92:345, 1969.

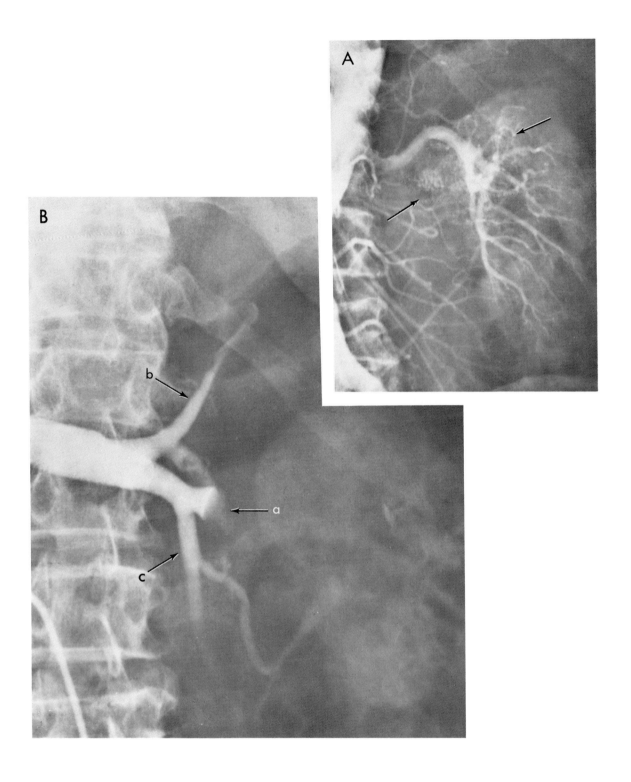

Figure 67 · Carcinoma: Renal Venography / 203

Figure 68.—Obstruction of the renal vein by tumor.

A, selective left renal arteriogram, arterial phase, anteroposterior view: Delineating many irregular, tortuous, neoplastic vessels in the upper pole of the kidney (**arrows**).

B, same study, nephrogram phase: The renal vein was never seen to fill. Venous drainage is principally through enlarged collateral veins, particularly the superior capsular vein (**arrow**). Dilated, tortuous pelvic and ureteral veins around the hilus (**a**) are responsible for notching of the ureter seen in the urogram.

A woman of 60 had a nodule on her scalp. Biopsy study proved it to be a metastatic carcinoma of renal origin.

Comment: The demonstration of dilated collateral veins draining the kidney with no visualization of the main renal vein on late films of the angiogram is a reliable (though not unequivocal) sign that the renal vein is completely or partially obstructed, presumably by tumor extension.* This finding can be brought out more clearly if selective angiography is performed with larger amounts of contrast agent (25 cc) after a diagnosis of renal malignancy has been obtained with routine dosages.

Figure 68, courtesy of Bosniak, M. A., O'Connor, J. F., and Caplan, L. H.: Renal arteriography in patients with metastatic renal cell carcinoma: Its use as a substitute for histopathologic biopsy, J.A.M.A. 203:249, 1968.

---

* Genereux, G. P.: The collateral vein sign in renal neoplasia, J. Canad. A. Radiologists 19:46, 1968.

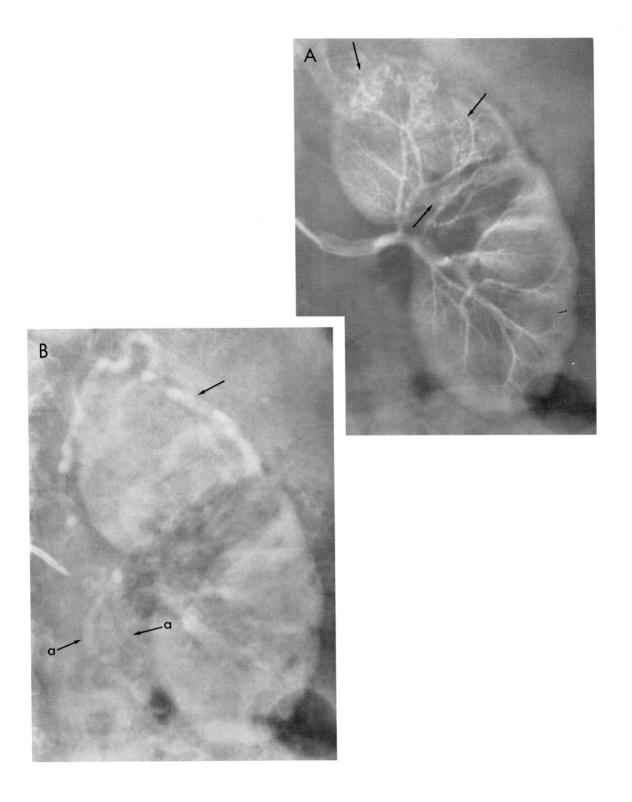

Figure 68 · Tumor Obstruction of Renal Vein / 205

Figure 69.—Renal carcinoma with extension to the adrenal gland.

A, selective right renal arteriogram, arterial phase, anteroposterior exposure: Revealing a huge vascular malignant lesion filling the right kidney. Note extension of tumor vessels into the adrenal gland at the upper pole of the kidney (**arrow**).

B, same study, nephrogram phase: Showing a well-defined adrenal gland

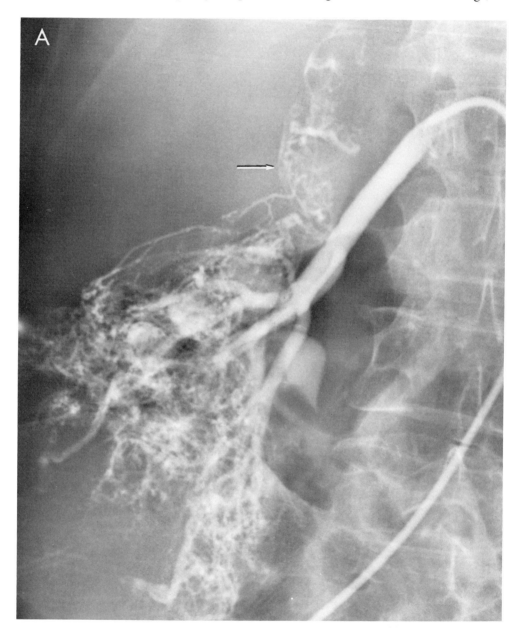

filled with tumor (**arrows**) as well as replacement of almost the entire kidney by tumor tissue.

A 64-year-old man with hematuria was hospitalized. An intravenous urogram disclosed a large mass in the right kidney. Right nephrectomy and adrenalectomy were performed for renal cell carcinoma of the kidney with involvement of the adrenal gland.

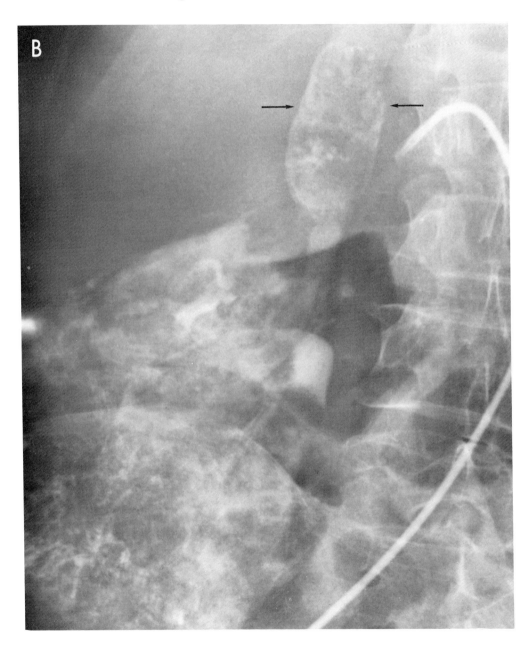

Figure 69 · Carcinoma Extension to the Adrenal / 207

Figure 70.—Angiographic demonstration of renal cell carcinoma metastatic to adjacent lymph nodes (same patient as in Fig. 66).

Selective right renal arteriogram, late arterial phase, anteroposterior exposure: Because the catheter tip is partly in the lumbar artery orifice, considerable opacification of retroperitoneal vessels as well as renal vessels has occurred. Intrarenal vessels show the typical appearance of renal cell carcinoma. Note the striate appearance of vessels overlying the upper pole and feeding extension of the tumor into the renal vein and vena cava (**arrow**; and see Fig. 65). Adjacent lymph nodes containing metastatic carcinoma are also well opacified (**a**).

This man of 46 had weakness and leg edema. Intravenous urography revealed a mass in the right kidney, and inferior venacavography demonstrated complete obstruction of the vena cava (Fig. 66). At surgery the tumor was found to have extended into the renal vein and the vena cava, and large nodes filled with tumor were identified at the kidney hilus.

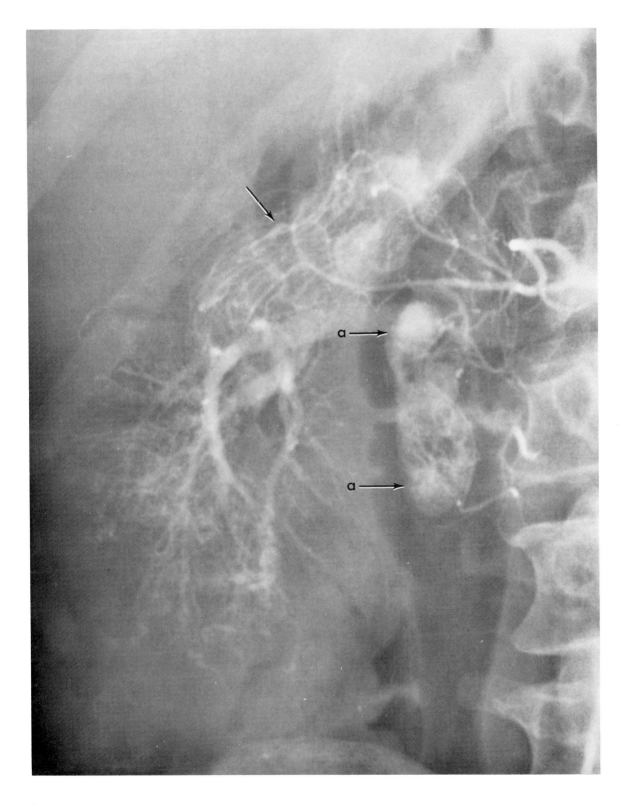

Figure 70 · Carcinoma: Lymph Node Metastasis / 209

Figure 71.—Carcinoma of the kidney with vascular metastasis to the spine.

A, intravenous urogram, anteroposterior projection: Showing a mass at the lower pole of the right kidney distorting the lower pole calyx (**arrows**). Note absence of the right pedicle of the fifth lumbar vertebra (**x**) and corresponding defect in the Pantopaque column from a previous myelogram.

(*Continued* on p. 212.)

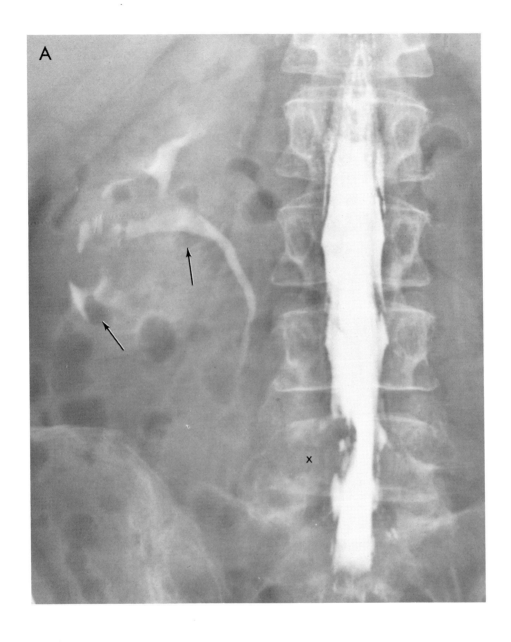

Figure 71 · Carcinoma: Spinal Metastasis / 211

Figure 71 (cont.).—Carcinoma of the kidney with vascular metastasis to the spine.

B, arteriogram, early phase, anteroposterior view: Demonstrating a large vascular neoplasm in the lower pole of the right kidney. There is hypertrophy of the fourth right lumbar artery (**arrow**), and increased vascularity in the region of the metastatic disease seen in **A.**

C, same study, nephrogram phase: Highlighting the metastasis to the fifth lumbar vertebra (**arrows**).

A woman of 68 was examined because of low back pain. A needle

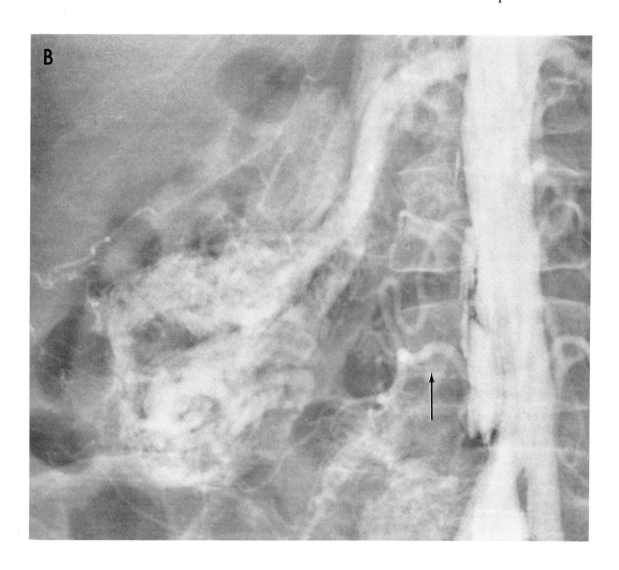

biopsy specimen from the fifth lumbar vertebra revealed "clear cell carcinoma." Radiotherapy was administered to the spine and the adjacent renal neoplasm.

Comment: The angiogram revealed the complete nature of this patient's disease. The primary lesion as well as the metastatic focus were delineated so that appropriate therapy could be instituted without delay. Angiography in such cases may be used as a substitute for histologic biopsy diagnosis.*

Figure 71, courtesy of Dr. B. L. Eisenberg, Suffern, N.Y.

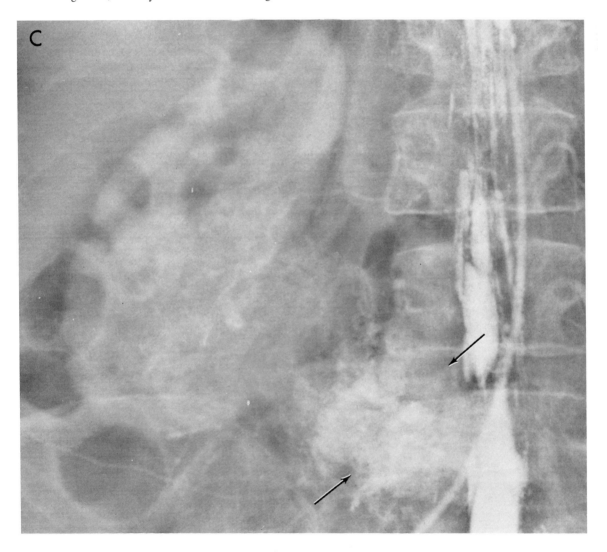

* Bosniak, M. A.; O'Connor, J. F., and Caplan, L. H.: Renal arteriography in patients with metastatic renal cell carcinoma: Its use as a substitute for histopathologic biopsy, J.A.M.A. 203:249, 1968.

Figure 71 · Carcinoma: Spinal Metastasis / 213

Figure 72.—Recurrent renal cell carcinoma in the kidney bed.

A, intravenous urogram, anteroposterior projection: Revealing increased density and a suggestion of a mass in the right flank. Enlargement of the left kidney is probably due to previous right nephrectomy.

B, aortogram, anteroposterior view: Demonstrating a large vascular tumor in the right renal bed. The tumor is fed by hypertrophied lumbar arteries (**arrows**), middle adrenal artery (**a**) and right spermatic artery (**b**).

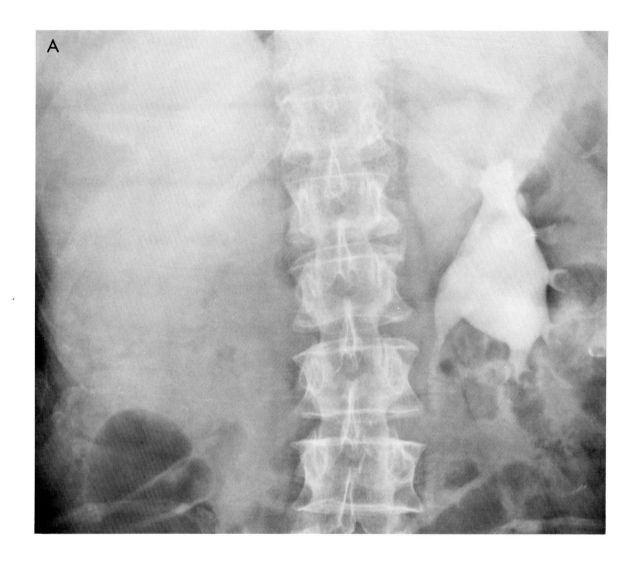

A 69-year-old man was hospitalized because of right flank pain. A right nephrectomy had been performed seven years previously for renal cell carcinoma. Following the studies shown here, the patient was not operated on but received radiotherapy to the tumor area, with some relief of symptoms. The angiogram in this case substituted for a histopathologic biopsy study and enabled therapy to be directed to the recurrent tumor without further surgery.

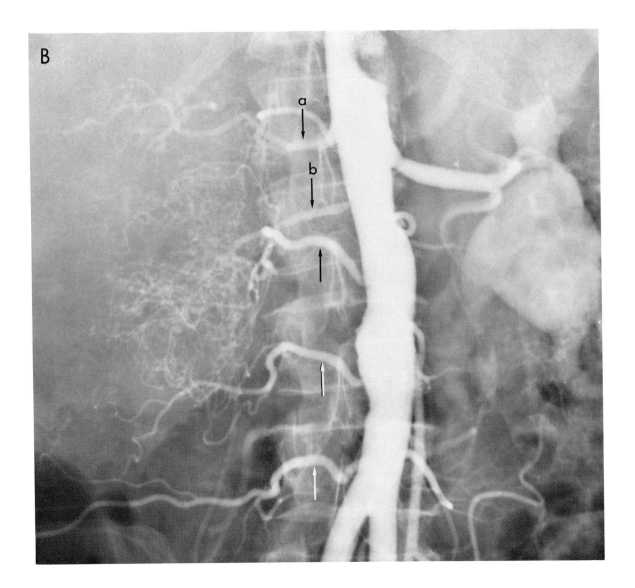

Figure 72 · Recurrent Carcinoma in Kidney Bed / 215

Figure 73.—Carcinoma of the kidney in a patient with Hippel-Lindau disease.

A, selective left renal arteriogram, arterial phase, anteroposterior projection: Revealing well-defined tumor vasculature in the midportion of the left kidney (**x**).

B, same study, nephrogram phase: Demonstrating the typical stasis and puddling of contrast medium in this malignant lesion (**x**).

A woman of 41 entered the hospital with neurologic symptoms. Family history revealed that five siblings had Hippel-Lindau disease, and the patient had clinical stigmas of this disease. An intravenous urogram revealed a left renal mass. At left nephrectomy a renal cell carcinoma was found.

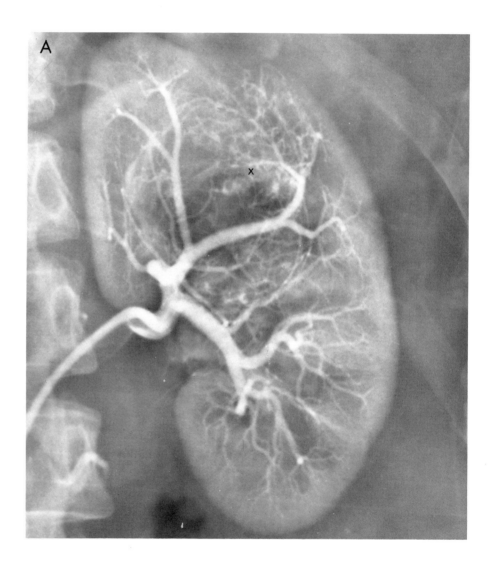

Comment: Either renal carcinoma or renal cysts, or both, may be present in two-thirds of patients with Hippel-Lindau disease. Because of this common association, patients with the disease should have frequent urologic observation. Renal angiography is indicated in all such patients when there is suspicion of a renal lesion.

Figure 73, courtesy of Dr. E. J. Ferris, Boston University Medical Center, Boston.

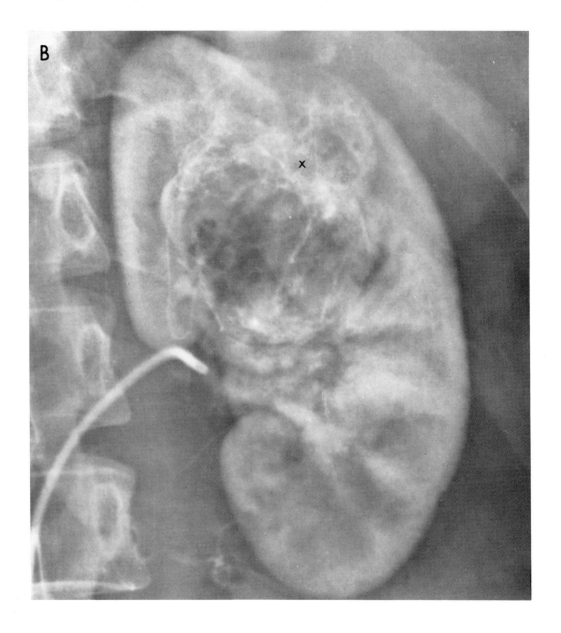

Figure 73 · Carcinoma with Hippel-Lindau Disease / 217

PART 4

*Malignancies of the Kidney
Parenchyma Other Than Carcinoma*

Clinical and Radiologic Characteristics

NONCARCINOMATOUS MALIGNANCIES of the kidney parenchyma include Wilms' tumor, mesenchymal tumors (including sarcoma), metastatic tumors to the kidney and lymphoma of the kidney. This is a heterogeneous group of lesions which obviously have varying clinical and radiologic characteristics. Although in most instances sarcomatous lesions cannot be differentiated from carcinoma, the other lesions in this group may have specific clinical and radiologic features that allow accurate diagnosis.

WILMS' TUMOR

Wilms' tumor, also called nephroblastoma, malignant nephroma, malignant embryoma and mesoblastic nephroma, constitutes about 6% of all renal cancers. It is rare in adults but is the second commonest abdominal tumor (after neuroblastoma) in the pediatric age group, accounting for about 20% of all tumors in childhood, whereas renal cancer constitutes 2–3% of all tumors in adults.

Wilms' tumor is considered to be an embryonic renal neoplasm containing a variety of tissues. Glandular and muscle elements predominate, but myxomatous tissue, fat and cartilage are also seen in this mixed neoplasm. The tumor probably develops from the metanephros.

About two-thirds of Wilms' tumors become manifest before 3 years of age. Children with sporadic aniridia and those with hemihypertrophy have a greater incidence of this tumor. Bilateral involvement is relatively rare, being reported in about 2% of the cases. Unlike children with neuroblastoma, most children with Wilms' tumor are asymptomatic. Over 50% have abdominal swelling or mass, 20–30% pain and only 5–10% hematuria.

Wilms' tumor spreads by direct extension but more commonly hematogenously, usually to the lung, sometimes to the liver and rarely to bone. Unfortunately 40–50% of children who are first seen after the age of 2 with this tumor have metastatic disease at the time of diagnosis. Only about 25% of children under 2 years of age have evidence of metastatic disease at the time of diagnosis, hence the better prognosis in the younger age group.

Intravenous urography is the basic roentgenologic study of a child with an abdominal mass. Wilms' tumor usually is seen as a large bulky flank mass on the abdominal roentgen examination. In the excretory urogram considerable distortion of the pelvocalyceal system is observed. The forms of distortion are varied and often cause bizarre calyceal patterns. Although there is no typical or pathognomonic deformity, dilatation, elongation and displacement of calyces are common findings. Some large tumors affect the collecting system only minimally, the kidney appearing to be displaced and attached to the periphery of the mass. In other instances the pelvis and calyces may be destroyed by tumor and the renal vein involved, causing nonvisualization urographically. In such cases differentiation from congenital hydronephrosis and multicystic kidney may not be possible on the urogram and further studies are necessary. Furthermore, it is not always possible on the basis of the anteroposterior projection of the urogram to decide whether the tumor is intrinsic to the kidney or primarily extrinsic. The lateral view is sometimes helpful to this decision and should be considered a routine part of the urographic examination (Fig. 75).

Inferior venacavography and angiography are sometimes used to advantage in studying children who present abdominal masses. Their application is demonstrated and discussed in Figures 76–78.

BIBLIOGRAPHY

Ackerman, L. V., and del Regato, J. A.: *Cancer* (3rd ed.; St. Louis: C. V. Mosby Company, 1962), p. 795.
Emmett, J. L.: *Clinical Urography* (2nd ed.; Philadelphia: W. B. Saunders Company, 1964), Vol. II, p. 805.
Nelson, W. E.; Vaughan, V., and McKay, R. J. (eds.): *Textbook of Pediatrics* (9th ed.; Philadelphia: W. B. Saunders Company, 1969), p. 1438.
Rubin, P.: Cancer of the urogenital tract: Wilms' tumor, J.A.M.A. 204:123, 1968.

MALIGNANT TUMORS OF MESENCHYMAL ORIGIN

This group of tumors, representing a large variety of histologic types, is fairly rare in the kidney, accounting for about 3% of all renal malignancies. For purposes of simplification we have included in this group almost all tumors of bizarre or unusual histology that will not fit into the other, more defined categories presented in this volume. The great majority of these tumors are sarcomas of various tissues of mesenchymal derivation. Many of them are of mixed mesenchymal origin and create considerable difficulty in specific labeling for the pathologist. Tumors included in this group are leiomyosarcomas, rhabdomyosarcomas, fibrosarcomas, osteogenic sarcomas, liposarcomas, angiosarcomas, hemangiopericytomas, mixed mesenchymal tumors including malignant angiomyolipomas, and various sarcomas of the capsule.

These tumors are usually indistinguishable radiologically from renal cell carcinoma. In the pyelogram they appear as masses in the kidney similar to renal cell carcinoma. Angiographic experience with these tumors is limited, but the angiogram usually correlates well with the predominant tissue in the tumor. For example, lesions with a large vascular component may be quite vascular, like an angiosarcoma, whereas less vascular tumors, like fibrosarcomas, may be quite hypovascular. In general, they cannot be distinguished from the wide range of vascularity of renal cell carcinomas. However, two radiographic findings are important in diagnosis. If the tumor contains large amounts of fat (e.g., liposarcoma and angiomyoliposarcoma) the mass may appear lucent on the routine films. Also, the bizarre vascular pattern of serpiginous, tortuous vessels with carcinoid aneurysms seen in angiomyolipomatous lesions (Figs. 83 and 97) apparently is characteristic of these tumors and may be helpful for histologic diagnosis.

BIBLIOGRAPHY

Lucké, B., and Schlumberger, H. G.: "Tumors of the Kidney, Renal Pelvis and Ureter"; Sec. VIII, Fasc. 30 of Armed Forces Institute of Pathology *Atlas of Tumor Pathology* (Washington, D.C.: 1957).

Turner-Warwick, R. T., and Thomson, A. D.: Connective Tissue and Mixed Tumours in Adults. In Riches, E. (ed.): *Tumours of the Kidney and Ureter* (Baltimore: Williams & Wilkins Company, 1964), p. 99.

METASTATIC NEOPLASMS TO THE KIDNEY

Neoplasms metastasize to the kidney either by direct extension or via the blood stream.

DIRECT EXTENSION.—Tumors of the renal pelvis, particularly squamous cell carcinomas, frequently extend into the kidney parenchyma (see Part 7, Tumors of the Renal Pelvis). Lymphoma, too, occasionally extends into the renal parenchyma from the retroperitoneal space (see discussion of lymphoma below). Very rarely, pararenal tumors such as pancreatic, adrenal and colon carcinomas extend into and invade the kidney.

BLOOD-BORNE METASTASES.—The blood-borne metastatic neoplasm to the kidney is a common autopsy finding but rarely is studied radiologically or clinically. Usually the metastases are small, multiple bilateral lesions. Occasionally, however, a single large focus does occur in the kidney, and this type of lesion can cause clinical symptoms and be demonstrated radiologically.

The kidney is the fifth most common site of metastases, after the liver, lung, bones and adrenals. Metastatic tumor to the kidney is more than twice as common as primary renal lesions. Tumors of the lungs and breast most often metastasize to the kidney, although renal metastases from primary tumors in all parts of the body have also been recorded.

RADIOGRAPHIC APPEARANCE.—Few cases of metastatic tumor to the kidney have been studied radiologically. Their pyelographic and angiographic appearance depends on the histology of the neoplasm and the extent of involvement. In our experience, squamous cell carcinomas have been invasive in character. Amputation and encasement of calyces and intrarenal vessels are seen with these tumors. A diminished nephrogram is also usual. There is little or no mass effect or tumor vasculature. Sarcomas and adenocarcinomas that we have studied have shown some similar characteristics but a less invasive quality. These lesions present as renal masses and display tumor vascularity angiographically, although the lesions have been generally hypovascular.

BIBLIOGRAPHY

Bosniak, M. A.; Stern, W.; Lopez, F.; Tehranian, N., and O'Connor, S. J.: Metastatic neoplasm to the kidney: A report of four cases studied with angiography and nephrotomography, Radiology 92:989, 1969.

Lucké, B., and Schlumberger, H. G.: "Tumors of the Kidney, Renal Pelvis and Ureter"; Sec. VIII, Fasc. 30 of Armed Forces Institute of Pathology *Atlas of Tumor Pathology* (Washington, D.C.: 1957).

Newsom, J. E., and Tulloch, W. S.: Metastatic tumours in the kidney, Brit. J. Urol. 38:1, 1966.

RENAL LYMPHOMA

Lymphoma of the kidneys is relatively rare and usually occurs late. Reticulum cell sarcoma and lymphosarcoma are more likely to involve the kidneys than Hodgkin's disease. The type of involvement of the kidney is quite variable and may be bilateral or unilateral. A localized single mass, multiple small parenchymal masses or diffuse infiltration of the kidney may occur. Occasionally, neoplastic invasion of the kidney by direct extension from pararenal retroperitoneal lymphoma is seen.

The pyelographic picture depends, of course, on the type of involvement. Swollen, enlarged kidneys with thickened cortex are seen when diffuse infiltration has occurred, whereas a picture not unlike that of polycystic kidneys may be observed when multiple lesions are present. Occasionally lymphoma will present as one large renal mass not unlike carcinoma. Renal displacement and obstruction with retroperitoneal lymphoma may occur.

The angiographic picture correlates well with the gross pathology. The vessels are stretched, pruned and encased by the infiltrating tumor tissue.

There are atrophy and decrease of terminal branching. A diminished nephrogram corresponds to the loss of renal tissue. This arterial pattern has been seen in the majority of reported cases and in our own experience, but tumor vascularity in this type of tumor has also been reported.

BIBLIOGRAPHY

Kyaw, M., and Koehler, P. R.: Renal and perirenal lymphoma: Arteriographic findings, Radiology 93:1055, 1969.

Lalli, A. F.: Lymphoma and the urinary tract, Radiology 93:1051, 1969.

Seltzer, R. A., and Wenlund, D. E.: Renal lymphoma: Arteriographic studies, Am. J. Roentgenol. 101:692, 1967.

Shapiro, J. H.; Ramsay, C. G.; Jacobson, H. G.; Bostein, C. C., and Allen, L. B.: Renal involvement in lymphomas and leukemias in adults, Am. J. Roentgenol. 88:928, 1962.

Watson, E. M.; Sauer, H. R., and Sadngor, M. G.: Manifestations of the lymphoblastomas in the genitourinary tract, J. Urol. 61:626, 1949.

Williams, L. H.; Anastopulos, H. P., and Presant, C. A.: Selective renal arteriography in Hodgkin's disease of the kidney, Radiology 93:1055, 1969.

Figure 74.—Wilms' tumor with metastases to the lungs.

A, intravenous urogram, anteroposterior projection: Showing a considerably enlarged right kidney. The bizarre configuration of the calyces and renal pelvis and their compression, elongation, separation and displacement are deformities typical of an intrarenal mass.

B, chest film, anteroposterior view: Revealing the lung fields studded with discrete round densities of varying size. This is the classic appearance of metastatic carcinoma in the lungs secondary to Wilms' tumor. The multiple

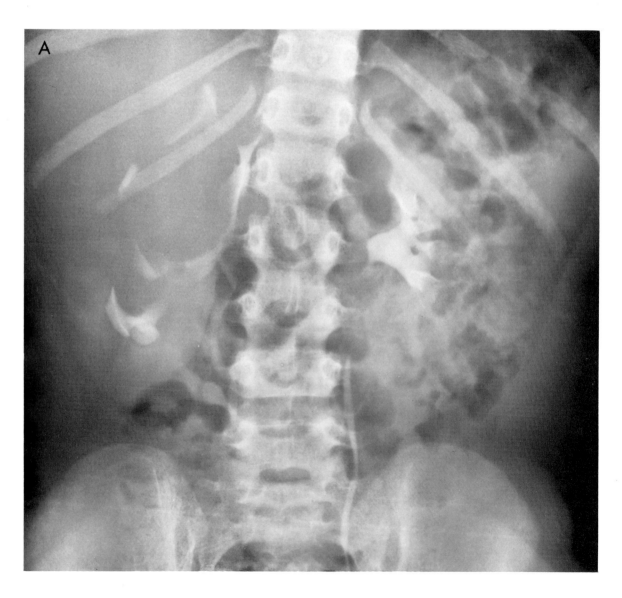

round masses, sometimes referred to as cannon balls or snowballs, are usually associated with blood-borne metastases to the lungs. This appearance is common with renal neoplasms because of their propensity to spread via the renal veins.

The patient, a 7-year-old girl, was found on a routine physical examination to have an abdominal mass.

Comment: The age, clinical data and destructive configuration of the collecting system on the urogram are all indicative of Wilms' tumor.

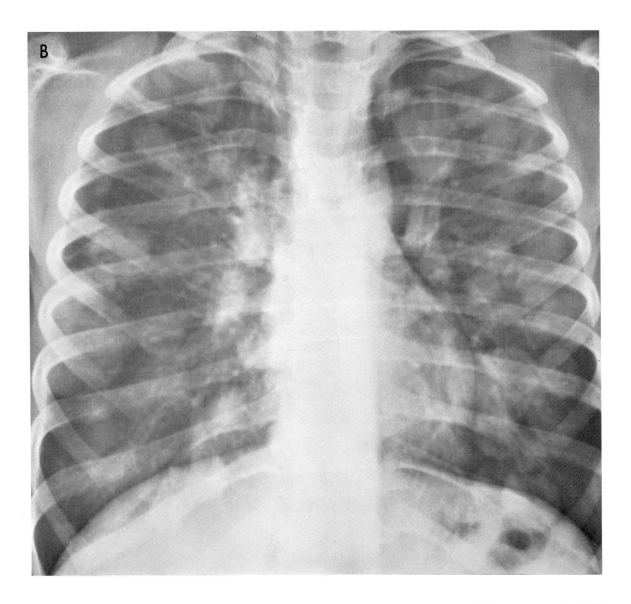

Figure 74 · Wilms' Tumor with Lung Metastases / 227

Figure 75.—Wilms' tumor with calcification.

A, intravenous urogram, anteroposterior exposure: Showing a huge left flank mass with irregular calcific deposits (**arrow**) which displaces the kidney and collecting system medially and inferiorly.

B, same study, lateral projection: Providing good appreciation of the dorsoventral extent of the mass. It also shows well the splaying, stretching and compression of the calyces characteristic of an intrarenal mass.

A 3½-year-old boy was hospitalized for investigation of a left flank mass. A left nephrectomy was performed. Pathologic diagnosis was nephroblastoma (Wilms' tumor) and radiotherapy was given.

Comment: Calcification in Wilms' tumor is quite unusual, being much more common in neuroblastoma. However, calcification can occur in any necrotic tissue. More important is whether the lesion is intrarenal or not. In this case the pronounced splaying of the calyces indicates that the lesion is clearly intrarenal and therefore a Wilms' tumor. The value of the lateral projection in demonstrating whether the tumor is intrarenal or extrarenal is evident.

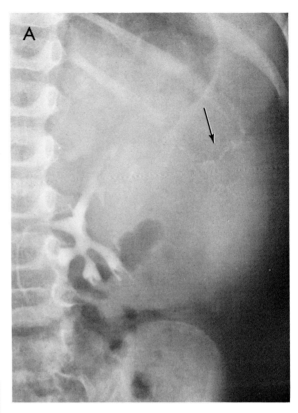

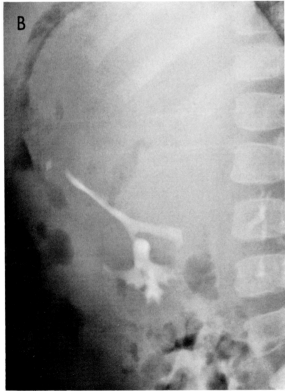

Figure 75 · Wilms' Tumor with Calcification / 229

Figure 76.—Wilms' tumor: inferior venacavography.

A, intravenous urogram, anteroposterior view: Showing a huge tumor occupying the whole right side of the abdomen. The entire collecting system of the right kidney is displaced medially and lies along the right border of the lumbar spine (**arrow**). The calyces are so stretched that they appear to lie in vertical tandem. Even though the collecting system seems to be on the medial periphery of the mass, the elongation, compression and splaying deformities indicate an intrarenal rather than extrarenal mass.

B, inferior venacavogram, with injection made via catheter in the left femoral vein, anteroposterior view: Demonstrating the poorly seen inferior vena cava (**arrows**) to be displaced medially, compressed and partially obstructed. Filling of collateral channels in the vertebral plexus and ascending lumbar vein (**a**) is clear.

A 7-month-old boy, born with hypospadias and chordee, was found during a routine physical examination to have an abdominal mass.

Comment: Inferior venacavography in a patient with Wilms' tumor provides the surgeon with important information regarding position, patency and presence of thrombus or tumor. Some pediatric radiologists believe this study should be routine in the investigation of such patients.* Intravenous urography can be accomplished by a needle inserted into a femoral vein, thus incorporating the inferior venacavogram as the initial phase of the urogram.

The technique is also useful in evaluating an infant with an abdominal mass and a nonfunctioning kidney demonstrated on urography. A patent cava in such a case suggests that the mass is probably benign, such as a multicystic kidney or hydronephrosis, whereas a blocked vena cava indicates Wilms' tumor.

---

* Hope, J. W.: Cancer of the urogenital tract: Radiographic differential diagnosis, J.A.M.A. 204:125, 1968.

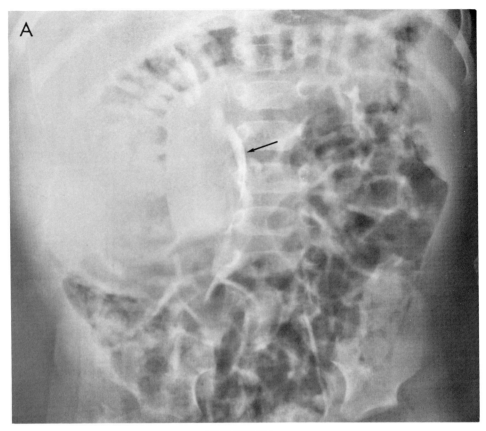

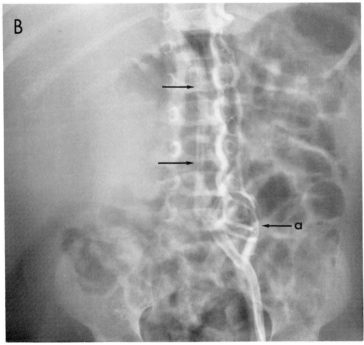

Figure 76 · Wilms' Tumor: Venacavography / 231

Figure 77.—Wilms' tumor: arteriography.

A, intravenous urogram, left posterior oblique projection: Revealing elongation, compression and splaying of the calyces of the left kidney, indicating an intrarenal mass.

B, selective left renal arteriogram, anteroposterior view: Showing the intrarenal vessels displaced by a large relatively hypovascular mass. A number of intrarenal arteries enter the mass, several of which have an abnormal appearance (**arrow**). Note also the hypertrophied capsular arteries feeding the neoplasm (**a**).

A boy of 8 entered the hospital with hematuria. He had had moderately severe trauma to the left flank a week previously. Left nephrectomy revealed nephroblastoma (Wilms' tumor).

Comment: Wilms' tumor in the infant and young child is usually readily diagnosed on the basis of clinical data and conventional urography. But in the older child, and particularly when the diagnosis is at all in doubt, arteriography is quite helpful. There is no specific arteriographic pattern for Wilms' tumor. Some are hypervascular, but most are hypovascular and exhibit few tumor vessels. The principal vascular effect may be vessel displacement with only minimal intrinsic vessel abnormality.*

In the case shown here, differential diagnosis on the basis of clinical data and urography included intrarenal hematoma and renal tumor. The angiogram established that the lesion was not a hematoma and probably was a renal tumor, although a large renal abscess may have the same arteriographic appearance. Renal arteriography therefore in certain circumstances has an important role in the diagnosis of Wilms' tumor.

---

* Meng, C. H., and Elkin, M.: Angiographic manifestations of Wilms' tumor: An observation of six cases, Am. J. Roentgenol. 105:95, 1969; McDonald, P., and Hiller, H. G.: Angiography in abdominal tumors with particular reference to neuroblastoma and Wilms' tumor, Clin. Radiol. 19:1, 1968.

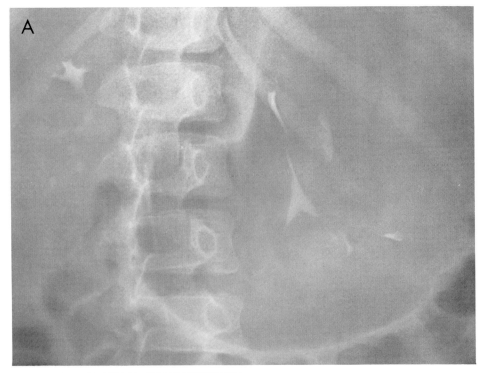

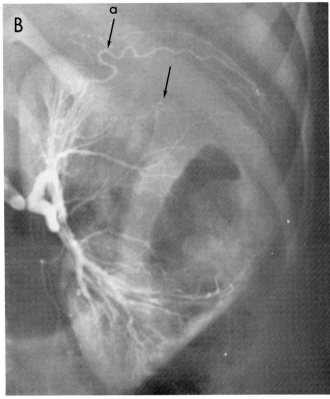

Figure 77 · Wilms' Tumor: Arteriography / 233

Figure 78.—Wilms' tumor: intravenous aortography.

A, right retrograde pyelogram, anteroposterior projection: Demonstrating a huge intrarenal mass involving the lower pole of the right kidney, with distortion, invasion and destruction of the collecting system. There is displacement of the ureter across the midline and inferior displacement of the colon.

(*Continued* on p. 236.)

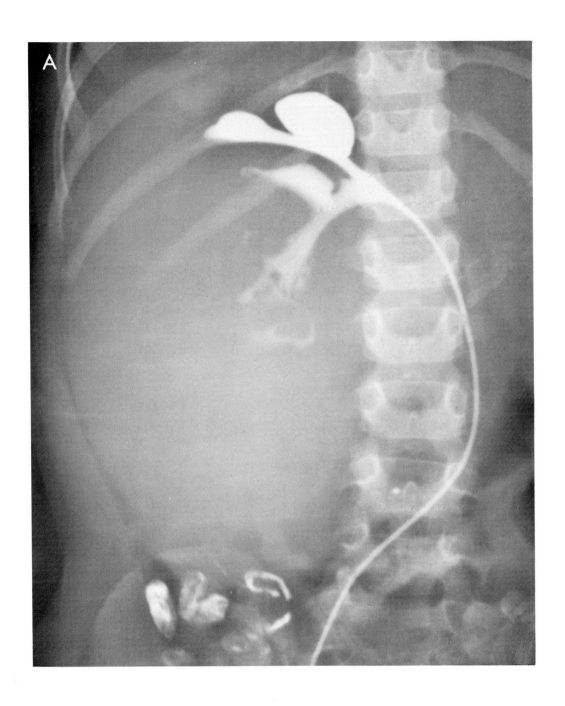

Figure 78 · Wilms' Tumor: Intravenous Aortography / 235

Figure 78 (cont.).—Wilms' tumor: intravenous aortography.

B, inferior venacavogram, anteroposterior view: Revealing medial displacement by the large right renal mass but no intrinsic defects. Radiolucency in the vena cava at the level of the renal veins represents return of nonopacified blood entering the vena cava from patent renal veins. There is also reflux into hepatic veins.

C, film obtained 12 seconds after **B,** revealing aortogram phase (see Comment): Showing faint but definite filling of the aorta (**x**) and its branches. The left kidney is normal. On the right, enlarged tortuous irregular tumor vessels are seen in the large renal tumor (**arrows**).

In a 4½-year-old girl with a right flank mass, intravenous urography showed poor visualization of the right kidney with a probable intrarenal

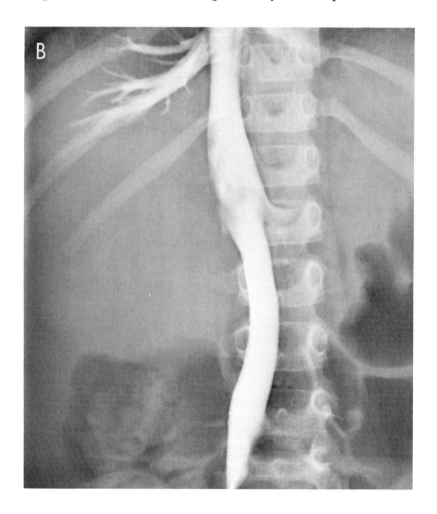

mass. Following the diagnosis of Wilms' tumor by the above described studies, preoperative radiotherapy was instituted, followed by right nephrectomy that revealed a well-encapsulated nephroblastoma (Wilms' tumor). The renal vein was free from tumor. Radiotherapy was then given to the tumor bed.

Comment: In this case the diagnosis was well established pyelographically because of the definite intrarenal location of the tumor shown by its effect on the collecting system. The cavogram was performed to rule out caval involvement to facilitate planning for surgery and radiotherapy. The aortogram was obtained by continuing the filming on a serial film-changer to include recirculation of the contrast medium to the aortic phase. The study, although done via the venous route, shows typical evidence of a malignant lesion in the right kidney. This technique can be used in small children when direct arteriography cannot be done. It does not have the diagnostic accuracy of selective arteriography but can be helpful in some instances.

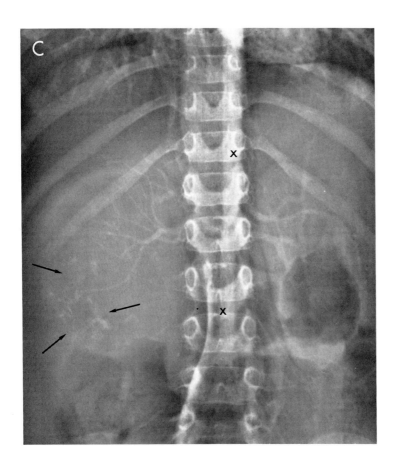

Figure 78 · Wilms' Tumor: Intravenous Aortography / 237

Figure 79.—Malignant mesenchymoma diagnosed with the aid of epinephrine angiography.

A, intravenous urogram, anteroposterior exposure: Showing slight displacement of the upper pole calyx (**arrow**).

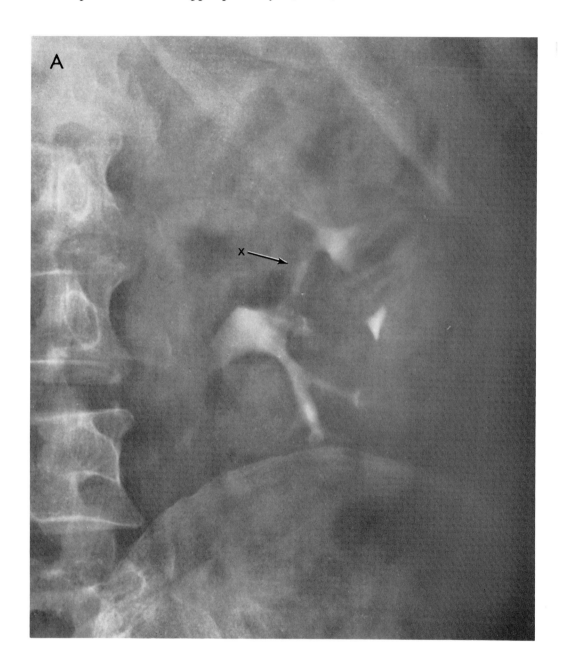

B, selective left renal arteriogram via the axillary artery, arterial phase, anteroposterior projection: Delineating stretched and attenuated vessels in the upper portion of the kidney and a decrease in the number of terminal branches in this area. No definite abnormal vessels are apparent, except possibly where a vessel extends too far peripherally (**arrow**).

(*Continued* on p. 240.)

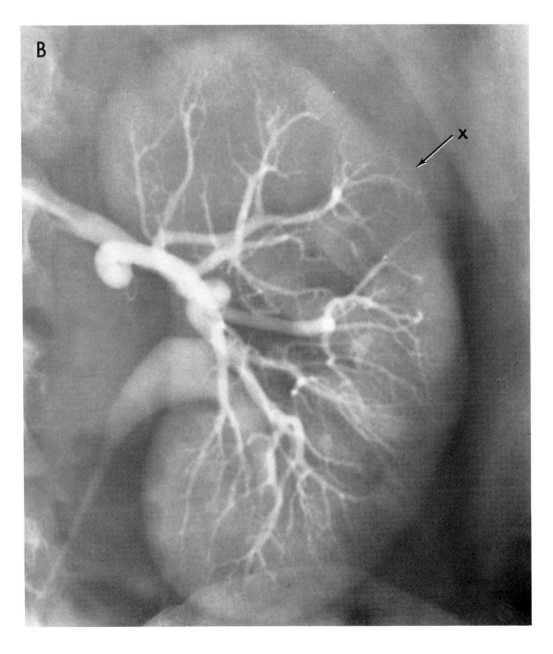

Figure 79 · Malignant Mesenchymoma / 239

Figure 79 (cont.).—Malignant mesenchymoma diagnosed with the aid of epinephrine angiography.

C, same study as **B,** nephrogram phase: Revealing loss of sharp contour of the kidney in the upper outer margin and stain outside the kidney (**a**). There is ill-defined radiolucency in the upper pole (**b**).

D, same study after instillation of 10 μg of epinephrine: Showing vessels to the lower portion of the kidney completely closed off; the vessels now visualized are not responding to epinephrine and have an abnormal appearance. The full extent of the malignancy at the upper pole of the left kidney is now outlined.

A man of 57, without symptoms relating to any organ symptom, was investigated because of 40 lb. weight loss which had begun a year previously. He had been well all his life. Left nephrectomy disclosed a large tumor occupying the posterior portion of the upper pole. At one point it had broken through the capsule and invaded the perinephric fat. The tumor was composed of fat, fibrous tissue, smooth muscle and neoplastic blood vessels and was thought to be a malignant mesenchymoma.

Comment: The exact histologic diagnosis in this case is open to question. Various pathologists might disagree with the final histologic interpretation, although they would agree that the lesion is a malignant sarcomatous tumor.

The case demonstrates the value of the epinephrine test. The standard angiogram shows only minimal changes indicative of the malignant nature of the lesion. The most important are the changes at the cortex seen in **C**. The epinephrine study established the diagnosis with more certainty and defined the extent of the lesion more accurately.

Figure 79, courtesy of Dr. Plinio Rossi, St. Vincent's Hospital, New York.

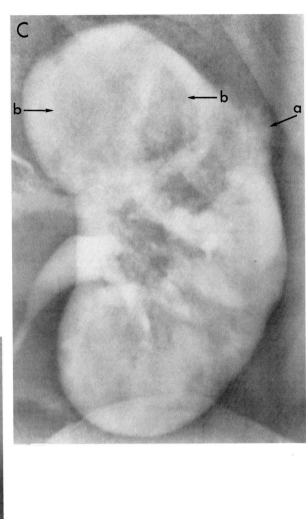

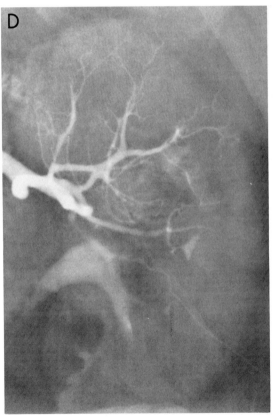

Figure 79 · Malignant Mesenchymoma / 241

Figure 80.—Spindle cell carcinoma of the left kidney.

A, left retrograde pyelogram, anteroposterior exposure: Showing poor definition of the upper pole of the left kidney and lateral rotation of the axis of the superior pole calyx.

B, selective left arteriogram, arterial phase, anteroposterior view: Revealing displacement of interlobar branches in the upper pole (**x**) and lack of normal filling and arborization of the small branches. There is loss of the upper pole nephrogram. Note separation of capsular and adrenal arteries from the kidney (**arrows**), indicating a perirenal process.

C, same study, nephrogram phase: Showing the apex of the upper pole to be deformed and its cortex irregular and somewhat ragged. A few small collections of contrast medium (**arrow**) suggest a localized tumor stain.

A woman of 42 had acute onset of left flank pain. An intravenous urogram revealed poor filling, concentration and visualization of the left pelvicalyceal system. At surgery a subcapsular hemorrhage and a necrotic mass involving the upper pole of the left kidney, was found and nephrectomy was performed. A number of pathologists who reviewed tissue sections differed as to whether the tumor was a spindle cell carcinoma or an extremely atypical angiomyolipoma.

Comment: In this case, the neoplasm at the upper pole of the kidney is poorly visualized. The more prominent findings are the separation of the adrenal and capsular vessels from the kidney indicating perirenal hematoma. We have seen a number of such cases in which small peripheral tumors of the kidney have presented clinically and radiologically as acute perirenal hematoma (see Fig. 40). The occurrence of such a circumstance should make one suspicious of an underlying neoplasm as a possible cause. (Other causes of acute perirenal hematoma include trauma, anticoagulation therapy, blood dyscrasias, periarteritis nodosa and vascular abnormalities.)

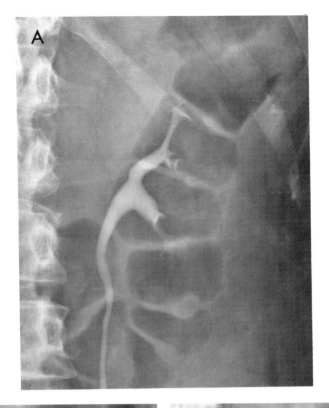

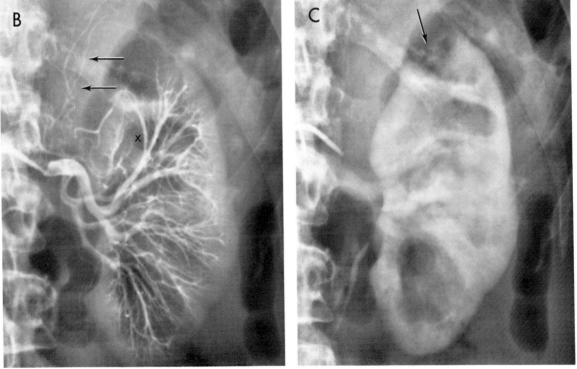

Figure 80 · Spindle Cell Carcinoma / 243

Figure 81.—Hemangiopericytoma of the right kidney.

A, intravenous urogram, anteroposterior projection: Showing the lower pole calyces of the right kidney draped over a mass located below the renal hilus.

B, selective right renal arteriogram (inferior accessory artery), anteroposterior view: Demonstrating a few vessels of abnormal appearance in the lower pole (**arrows**).

C, flush aortogram, nephrogram phase: Revealing a well-circumscribed vascular tumor stain (**arrows**) in the medial quadrant of the lower pole.

A woman of 31 complained of right flank pain. Examination disclosed nothing remarkable except microscopic pyuria and albuminuria. A right nephrectomy was performed. Histologic diagnosis was hemangiopericytoma.

Comment: The histopathologic diagnosis in this case was not clear cut. The sections were initially seen by a well-known tumor pathologist who made the diagnosis of low-grade hemangiopericytoma. They were later reviewed by another recognized tumor pathologist who made the diagnosis of benign hamartoma. This emphasizes the conflicting opinions that exist among pathologists with respect to the histology of certain tumors. This is particularly apt to be true among mesenchymal tumors. Radiologically the lesion does not appear to be a hamartoma (angiomyolipoma; see Figs. 96 and 97) but cannot be differentiated from a hypovascular renal cell carcinoma.

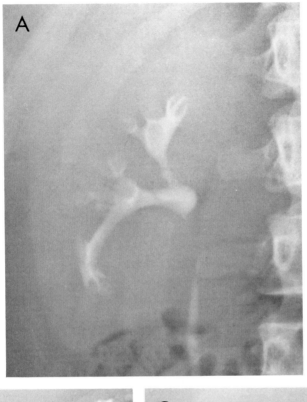

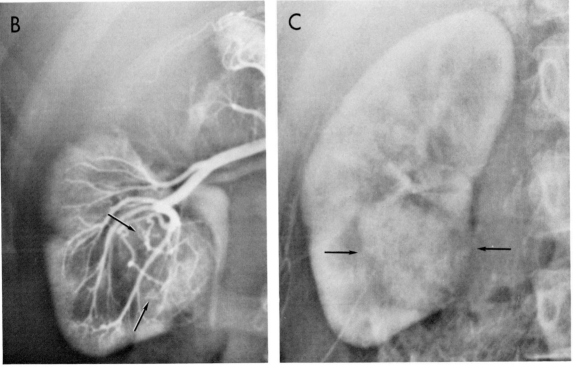

Figure 81 · Hemangiopericytoma / 245

Figure 82.—Malignant hemangiopericytoma of the right kidney.

Intravenous urogram, anteroposterior projection: Demonstrating displacement of the right kidney and ureter inferiorly and laterally by a large mass which involves the upper half of the kidney. The major portion of the mass is extrarenal. A small fleck of calcium is seen just medial to the renal pelvis (**arrow**). Note the biopsy site at **x**.

A 29-year-old woman had been well until she noted pain over the right ilium. An osteolytic lesion of the ilium was reported on biopsy examination to represent a hemangiopericytoma. Nephrectomy and partial ureterectomy were performed. The kidney weighed 700 g. Arising in the kidney was a $10 \times 10 \times 7.5$ cm, partially cystic and necrotic lobulated and malignant hemangiopericytoma which infiltrated the peripelvic tissues.

Comment: Hemangiopericytoma is an uncommon vascular tumor of relatively low malignancy. Its chief cellular component is the pericyte, a modified smooth muscle cell closely applied to the capillary wall and serving as regulator of the size of the capillary lumen. The tumor occurs in both sexes and at all ages from the neonatal period to senescence, but with a predilection for the middle decades. It has a wide distribution throughout the body. Renal involvement is quite rare, with few cases reported.* Calcification, which may be present within the tumor, often suggests angiosarcoma.

Figure 82, courtesy of Dr. D. M. Witten, Mayo Clinic, Rochester, Minn.

---

* Mujahed, Z.; Vasilas, A., and Evans, J. A.: Hemangiopericytoma: A report of four cases with a review of the literature, Am. J. Roentgenol. 82:638, 1959.

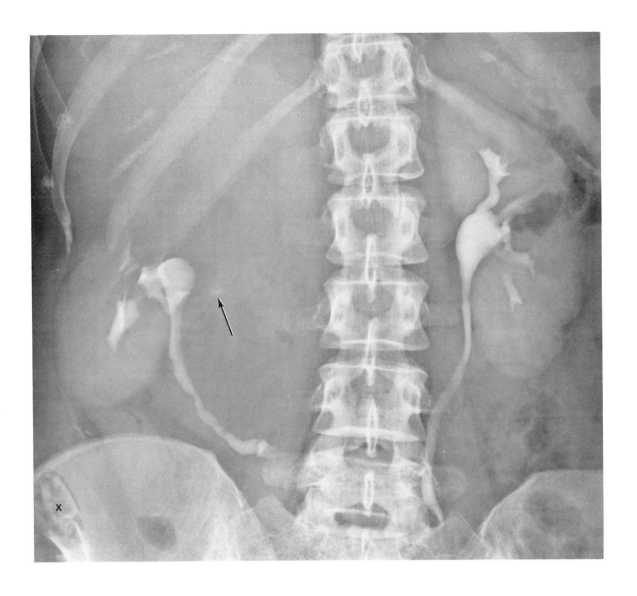

Figure 82 · Malignant Hemangiopericytoma / 247

Figure 83.—Bilateral malignant angiomyolipomas.

A, intravenous urogram, anteroposterior projection: Revealing a large mass at the lower pole of the left kidney (**arrows**) which displaces the inferior calyx superiorly and presses on the inferior margin of the renal pelvis. No definite abnormality of the right kidney can be seen.

(*Continued* on p. 250.)

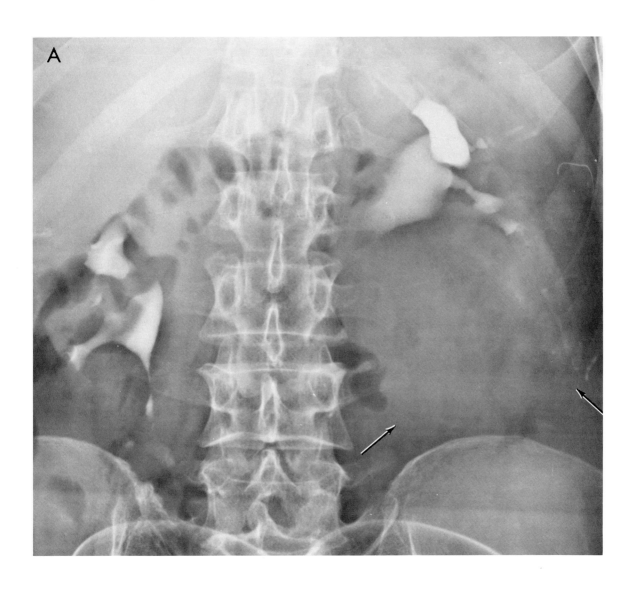

Figure 83 · Bilateral Malignant Angiomyolipomas / 249

Figure 83 (cont.).—Bilateral malignant angiomyolipomas.

B, selective left renal arteriogram, late arterial phase, anteroposterior view: Demonstrating a collection of abnormal-appearing vessels at the lower pole of the kidney. They are saccular and circinoid, with stasis and slow flow of contrast agent through them. The nephrogram phase is already present in the rest of the kidney.

C, selective right renal arteriogram, late arterial phase: Revealing a similar but smaller lesion on the lateral aspect of the right kidney.

A man of 55 was examined because of a left upper quadrant mass. On left renal exploration a biopsy specimen was obtained. The histologic diagnosis was unclear, with three different possibilities offered: malignant angiomyolipoma, leiomyosarcoma and a spindle cell variety of hypernephroid carcinoma. Chemotherapy was given and the patient was well a year later.

Comment: This case demonstrates two important points. The first is the importance of angiography in evaluating the opposite kidney when a nephrectomy is contemplated. The lesion in the right kidney cannot be fully appreciated in the intravenous urogram but is well demonstrated angiographically. The treatment plan was then changed from left nephrectomy to biopsy of the left lesion for purposes of selecting chemotherapy. Whether each lesion is an independent malignancy or the right kidney lesion is a metastasis from the left tumor is not certain. The case also points out the difficulties encountered by pathologists in putting a definite histologic name to some bizarre sarcomatous lesions. On the basis of the angiographic appearance, we believe that we are dealing with an angiomyolipoma (see Figs. 96 and 97).

Figure 83, courtesy of Drs. J. J. Bookstein and A. F. Lalli, Ann Arbor, Mich.

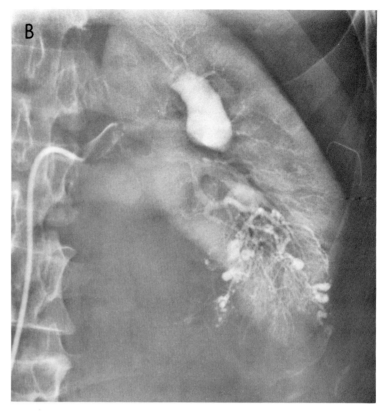

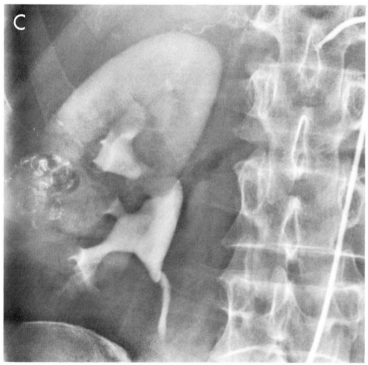

Figure 83 · Bilateral Malignant Angiomyolipomas / 251

Figure 84.—Fibrosarcoma of the renal capsule.

A, intravenous urogram, anteroposterior projection: Revealing a large suprarenal mass that displaces and rotates the left kidney.

B, nephrotomogram, anteroposterior view: Showing the opacified mass, indicating that it is vascular (**arrows**). The renal margin (**a**) is clearly visible, indicating that the lesion is extrarenal though adjacent to the kidney. From this study, a diagnosis of adrenal or pararenal tumor might be made.

(*Continued* on p. 254.)

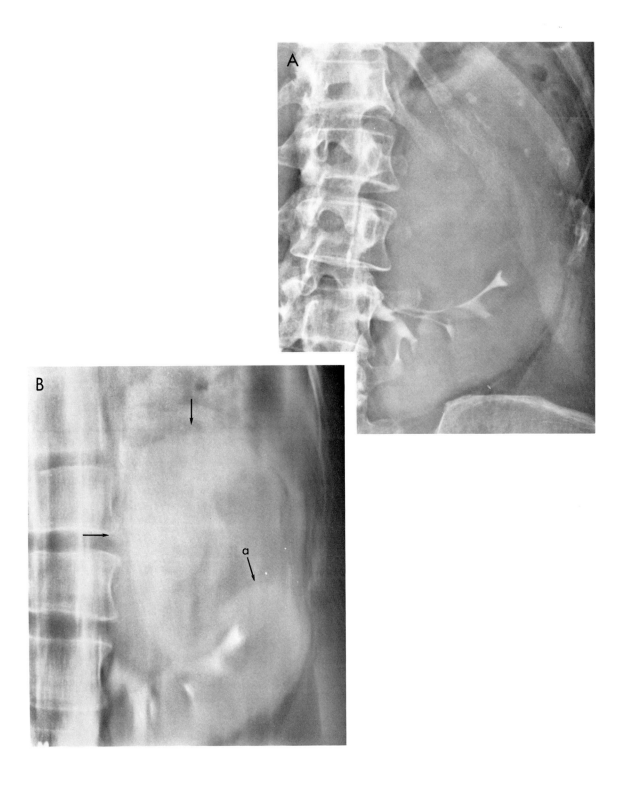

Figure 84 · Fibrosarcoma of Renal Capsule / 253

Figure 84 (cont.).—Fibrosarcoma of the renal capsule.

C, selective left renal arteriogram, anteroposterior view: Showing the main renal artery and kidney displaced inferiorly by the mass. The lesion is fed mainly by adrenal and capsular arteries (**arrows**) and a few small branches from the main renal artery. Numerous thin irregular tortuous vessels course throughout and along the periphery of the mass. No perforating renal arteries are seen extending into the tumor, which appears to be extrarenal, suggesting a diagnosis of suprarenal or pararenal neoplasm.

A woman of 61 had hematuria. At surgery the mass appeared to be contiguous with the kidney and could not be physically separated from the renal substance. A radical left nephrectomy was performed. The pathologic report indicated a fibrosarcoma most likely arising from the renal capsule.

Comment: Tumors of the renal capsule are basically extrarenal lesions and sometimes are grouped with retroperitoneal tumors. Because of the intimate connection of the kidney and its capsule, most tumors of the capsule get renal as well as capsular blood supply. In this instance, the major blood supply was seen originating from capsular arteries, suggesting the diagnosis of extrarenal neoplasm. Since the lesion was suprarenal in location in this case, the possibility of an adrenal neoplasm was also considered.

Renal capsule tumors are quite rare. Most malignant tumors of the capsule are fibrosarcomas, but leiomyosarcomas and liposarcomas have also been described.

Figure 84, courtesy of Dr. J. A. Becker, State University of New York, Downstate Medical Center, Brooklyn, New York.

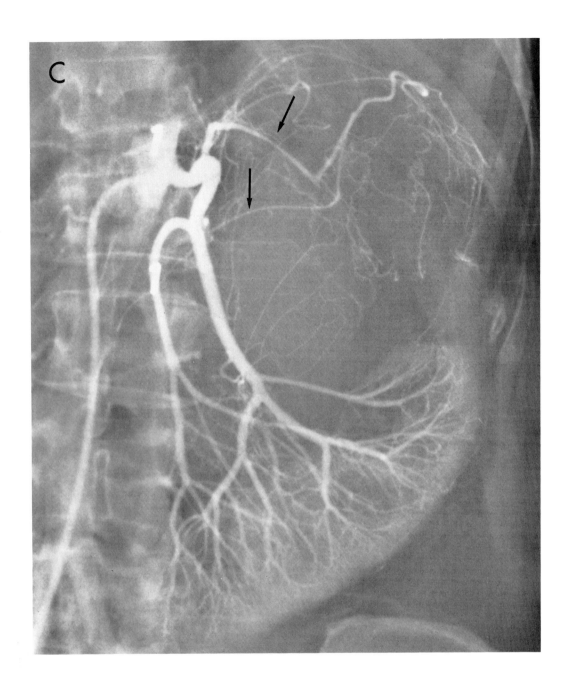

Figure 84 · **Fibrosarcoma of Renal Capsule** / 255

Figure 85.—Metastasis to the kidney from squamous cell carcinoma of the lung.

A, left retrograde pyelogram, anteroposterior projection: Showing that the calyces in the lower pole of the left kidney cannot be filled.

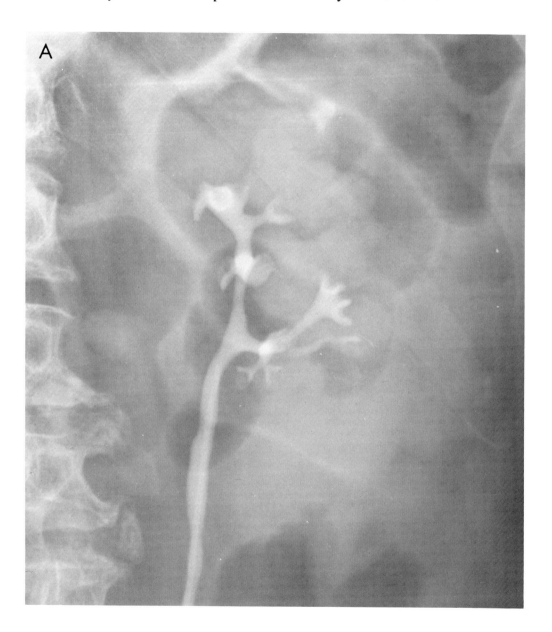

B, selective left renal arteriogram, early phase, anteroposterior view: Demonstrating diminished vascularity in the lower pole of the kidney. The irregularity of vessels in the lower pole (**arrows**) indicates tumor encasement.

(*Continued* on p. 258.)

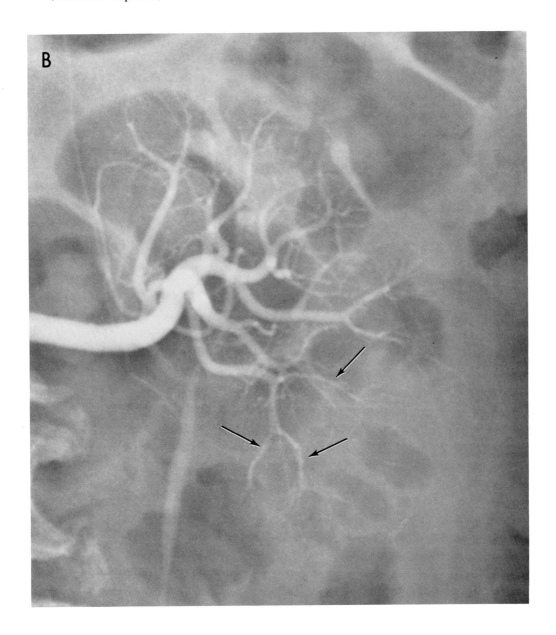

Figure 85 · Metastases from Lung / 257

Figure 85 (cont.).—Metastasis to the kidney from squamous cell carcinoma of the lung.

C, same study as **B,** late phase: Delineating no tumor vessels, but a slow flow of contrast medium through the lower pole arteries. Note that the vessels are encased, as manifested by irregular narrowing and amputation (**arrows**). A decreased number of terminal branches is observed and there is a diminished nephrogram throughout the lower pole.

D, surgical specimen: Showing the lower pole of the kidney replaced by epidermoid carcinoma metastatic from the lung.

A man of 59 was hospitalized because of left flank pain. He had received radiotherapy for epidermoid carcinoma of the lung seven months previously. Intravenous urography demonstrated poor visualization of the lower pole of the left kidney. Left nephrectomy was performed.

Comment: Usually, metastatic carcinoma to the kidney is an incidental finding at autopsy and rarely causes symptoms. Occasionally, however, a single large metastasis develops in the kidney and may cause symptoms and radiologic signs, as in this case. Metastatic lesions that have proved to be squamous cell carcinoma have shown a similar pattern (as seen in this case) —encasement of structures (vessels, calyces) by tumor (see also Fig. 86). The pattern may be characteristic enough so that in the proper clinical setting the diagnosis of metastatic carcinoma to the kidney can be made, thereby obviating the need for exploratory surgery (see Bosniak *et al.* below).

Figure 85, courtesy of Bosniak, M. A.; Stern, W.; Lopez, F.; Tehranian, N., and O'Connor, S. J.: Metastatic neoplasm to the kidney: A report of four cases studied with angiography and nephrotomography, Radiology 92:989, 1969.

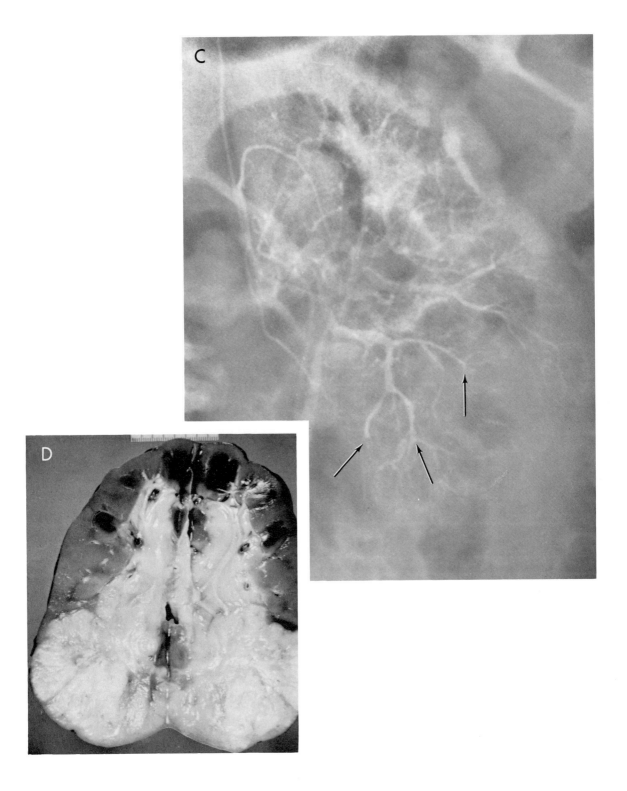

Figure 85 · Metastases from Lung / 259

Figure 86.—Metastasis to the kidney from squamous cell carcinoma of the esophagus.

Selective left renal arteriogram, anteroposterior projection: Showing vessels to the lower pole to be poorly filled. Many appear to be amputated. Small capsular vessels extend along the kidney margin. The nephrogram in the lower pole is lacking, in contrast to a well-visualized nephrogram in the upper pole.

A 52-year-old man was hospitalized because of painless hematuria. Three years previously he had undergone esophagectomy and esophagogastrostomy for carcinoma of the esophagus, followed by radiotherapy. An intravenous urogram now revealed nonfilling of the lower pole calyx of the left kidney. At left nephrectomy, squamous cell carcinoma identical to the previously removed esophageal carcinoma was found, involving the lower pole of the kidney.

Comment: The findings are typical of squamous cell carcinoma metastatic to the kidney. The tumor infiltrated and replaced normal renal tissue, with resulting vessel encasement and truncation. Calyceal structures as well as vessels may be involved, and the nephrogram is diminished.

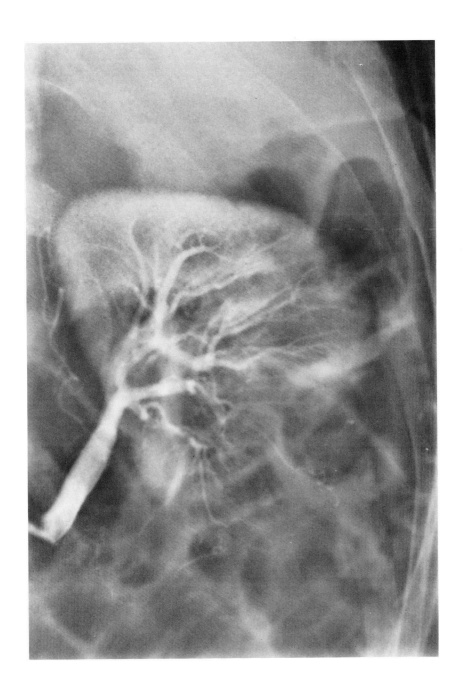

Figure 86 · Metastases from Esophagus / 261

Figure 87.—Burkitt's tumor of the kidney.

Intravenous urogram, anteroposterior projection: Demonstrating enlargement of the upper and lateral portions of the left kidney with associated calyceal distortion of the upper pole calyceal group.

A 10-year-old boy had Burkitt's tumor of multiple areas of the body.

Comment: Burkitt's tumor is a poorly differentiated lymphocytic lymphoma containing nonmalignant histiocytes. The condition is often multifocal and may be present with bone tumors (the jaw is frequently involved) and/or with multiple visceral tumors, particularly of the liver, kidneys and adrenals. When the kidneys are involved the urographic pattern is similar to that described for lymphoma with a varied pattern of involvement. The most common presentation would be that of multiple renal masses. The condition, which occurs principally in parts of Africa, presents in patients before puberty and rarely over the age of 20 years.

Figure 87, courtesy of Whittaker, L. R.: Intravenous pyelography in Burkitt's tumour, Australasian Radiol. 14: 197, 1970.

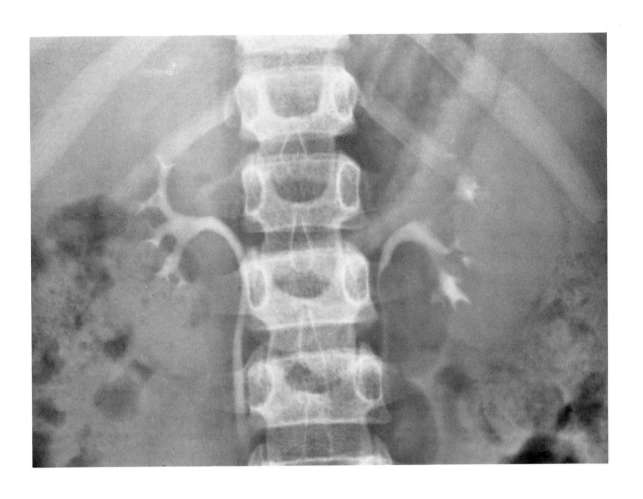

Figure 87 · Burkitt's Tumor of the Kidney / 263

Figure 88.—Lymphoma (reticulum cell sarcoma) of the kidney.

A, right retrograde pyelogram, anteroposterior projection: Revealing encasement of the upper ureter, renal pelvis and middle and lower pole infundibular structures by tumor. The upper calyces are hydronephrotic.

B, selective right renal arteriogram, anteroposterior exposure: Showing stretching, attenuation, encasement and truncation of vessels, most marked in the middle and lower segments of the kidney. The nephrogram is also poor in these areas. The localized hydronephrosis of the upper pole calyces results in some stretching, but encasement is not present, and loss of the nephrogram is not as great as elsewhere.

A 30-year-old man, who had had laparotomy and diagnosis of reticulum cell sarcoma in the retroperitoneal space, was hospitalized for evaluation of loss of renal function on the right. On intravenous urography the right kidney could not be visualized.

Comment: Attenuation, encasement and truncation of the vessels is a vascular pattern that is produced by a diffusely infiltrating lesion and is commonly seen in metastatic carcinoma (squamous cell) to the kidney and in renal pelvic tumors when they infiltrate the renal parenchyma (see Figs. 120 and 121), as well as lymphoma. The findings in the lower two-thirds of the kidney in this case are quite similar to those in Figure 89 and to those described in the literature.

Figure 88, courtesy of Dr. Ervin Philipps, Woodland, Calif.

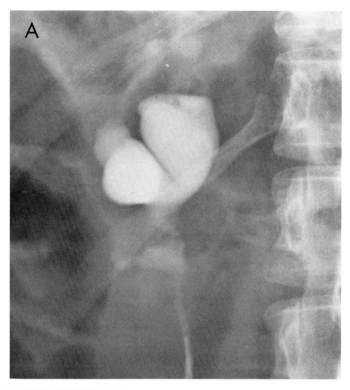

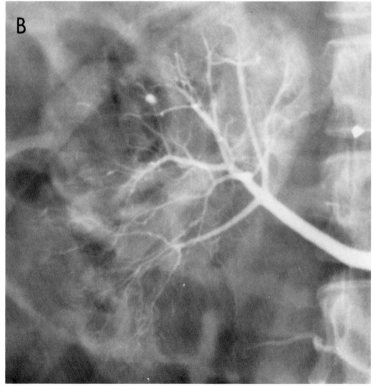

Figure 88 · Lymphoma (Reticulum Cell Sarcoma) / 265

Figure 89.—Reticulum cell sarcoma involving both kidneys.

A, selective right renal arteriogram, anteroposterior projection: Delineating small renal vessels as compared to the large size of the kidney. Intrarenal arteries are stretched and attenuated. There is poor filling of terminal branches, and the nephrogram is diminished and spotty.

B, selective left renal arteriogram: Showing an arteriographic pattern similar to that of the right kidney (**A**). The vessels have a thin, stretched appearance due to encasement by a diffuse lymphomatous infiltrate.

C, abdominal film 24 hours after arteriography: Demonstrating the large size (14.0 cm) of both kidneys (**arrows**). The spotty nephrogram is due to decreased renal function secondary to lymphomatous infiltration and replacement of renal tissue.

An 8-year-old boy entered the hospital with hypertension. He was known to have reticulum cell sarcoma, proved by bone biopsy. Intravenous urography revealed large kidneys but no visualization of the collecting system.

Comment: The large poorly functioning kidneys are characteristic of diffuse lymphomatous involvement as shown in this case. Other conditions that can cause bilaterally enlarged, poorly functioning kidneys include diseases that infiltrate the kidney (leukemia, amyloidosis, von Gierke's disease), conditions that obstruct the kidneys (hydronephrosis and renal vein thrombosis), bilateral tumors (polycystic kidneys) and conditions causing edema of the kidney (acute pyelonephritis, acute glomerulonephritis and nephrosis).

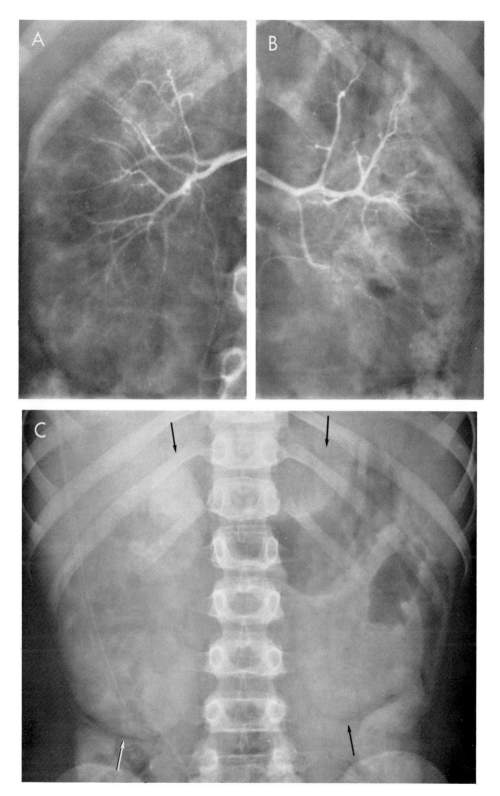

Figure 89 · Bilateral Reticulum Cell Sarcoma / 267

Figure 90.—Reticulum cell sarcoma.

A, intravenous urogram, anteroposterior exposure: Showing the left kidney to be somewhat enlarged but retaining its normal contour. There are distortion and compression of the upper and lower pole infundibula. The middle calyx is absent and appears to have been amputated by the infiltrating tumor. The renal pelvis also appears to be compressed and partially involved.

B, aortotomogram (tomogram taken during intravenous aortogram): Revealing the parenchyma in the midportion of the kidney has been replaced by a diffuse infiltrating mass, which results in a poor and spotty nephrogram. Renal and splenic arteries are seen **(arrows).**

A girl of 18 had a three month history of left flank and costovertebral pain followed by episodes of hemoptysis. The chest film revealed disseminated pulmonary metastases. The left kidney weighed 276 g. In its midportion was a 7×6×5 cm reticulum cell sarcoma which had invaded the renal pelvis and renal vein.

Comment: The generally poor nephrogram with loss of cortical definition and the apparent encasement of calyces with loss of the middle calyx and partial amputation of the renal pelvis are findings seen in malignant lymphoma.

Figure 90, courtesy of Dr. D. M. Witten, Mayo Clinic, Rochester, Minn.

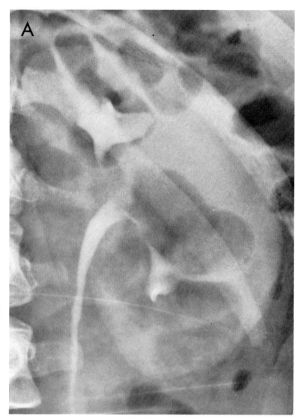

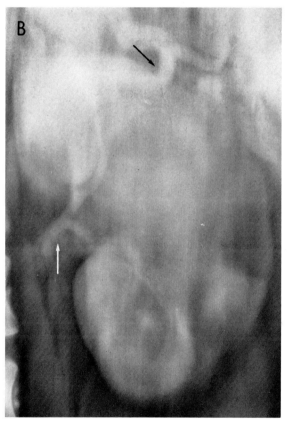

Figure 90 · Reticulum Cell Sarcoma / 269

Figure 91.—Reticulum cell sarcoma of the left kidney (intra- and extrarenal).

A, intravenous urogram, anteroposterior projection: Demonstrating lateral displacement of the left kidney by a large mass which has effaced most of the renal outline. The infundibula of the upper and middle calyceal groups are elongated and narrowed. The proximal ureter is also narrowed and displaced and suggests tumor encroachment.

B, nephrotomogram, aortotomogram phase, anteroposterior view: This examination was done by the original rapid intravenous injection technique. The aorta and renal arteries are well filled. The aorta is atherosclerotic. The left renal artery (**arrow**) and a few of the major intrarenal branches have the typical appearance of vascular encasement by tumor. There are loss of the psoas outline and complete loss of the renal borders except along the lateral margin. The appearance is that of a tumor of the perirenal tissue extending into the kidney sinus and parenchyma.

A 64-year-old woman was hospitalized because of left flank pain and weight loss. At surgery the left kidney was judged to be inoperable; a biopsy specimen revealed reticulum cell sarcoma.

Comment: In this instance the lymphomatous process involved the retroperitoneal space and extended directly into the renal sinus and parenchyma.

Figure 91, courtesy of Dr. D. M. Witten, Mayo Clinic, Rochester, Minn.

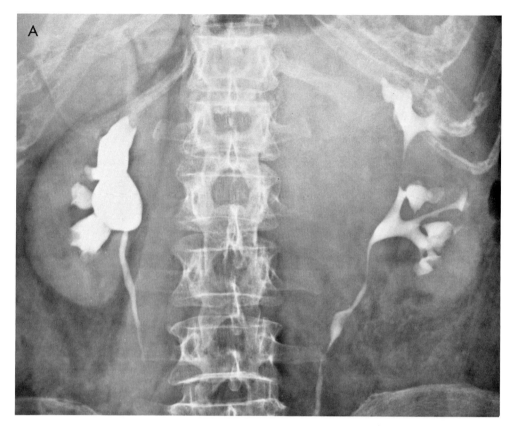

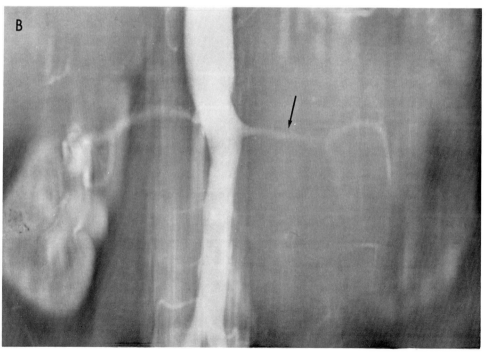

Figure 91 · Reticulum Cell Sarcoma (Intra- & Extrarenal) / 271

Figure 91–1.—Lymphoma (giant follicular) of the kidney.

A, intravenous urogram, anteroposterior projection: Showing enlargement of the right kidney (17.0 cm) with thickening of the parenchyma and stretching of the infundibular structures, particularly in the upper portions (**arrow**). The left kidney measured 12 cm.

B, selective right renal arteriogram, anteroposterior view: Revealing stretching of vessels with decreased filling of terminal branches at the upper pole where the kidney margin is indistinct and the nephrogram is not present. There is iatrogenic embolization of a lower pole vessel (**arrow**). No pathologic vessels are apparent.

The patient was a 59-year-old woman who had had a diagnosis of giant follicular lymphoma for 13 years.

Comment: The lymphoma involved only the right kidney, particularly the upper portion. Lymphoma is usually an infiltrative disease in the kidney and replaces normal parenchyma, which explains the radiographic findings —enlargement of the kidney, attenuation and narrowing of infundibular and arterial structures and diminished nephrogram.

Figure 91–1, courtesy of Dr. Ervin Philipps, Woodland, Calif.

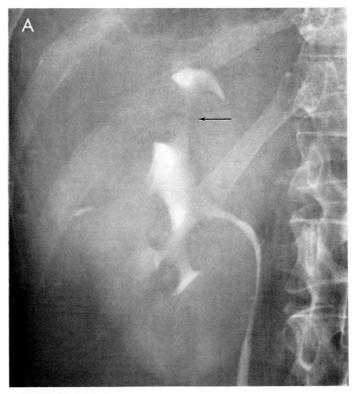

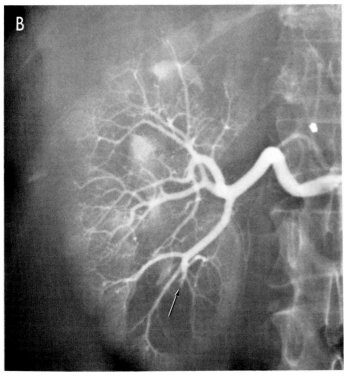

Figure 91–1 · Lymphoma (Giant Follicular) of the Kidney / 273

PART 5

Benign Tumors of the Kidney Parenchyma

General Characteristics of Benign Parenchymal Tumors

BENIGN PARENCHYMAL tumors of the kidney consist of adenomas (renal cell tumors) and mesenchymal tumors (connective tissue tumors). The mesenchymal tumors include fibromas, myomas, lipomas, angiomas and mixed mesenchymal tumors (angiolipomas). The great majority of these benign tumors are quite small, and usually are not studied clinically but are found incidentally at autopsy. On occasion, however, one attains a considerable size, causes symptoms and can be studied radiographically. Our experience with these benign tumors has been limited to adenoma, hemangioma, lipoma and angiomyolipoma; therefore the discussion and illustrative radiologic observations include only these lesions.

ADENOMA

Adenomas of the kidney are small nodules usually less than 1 cm in size. They are frequently multiple, are found in the cortex usually beneath the capsule and ordinarily are discovered incidentally at autopsy. Occasionally, but rarely, they are larger, reaching a diameter of 3–4 cm. These larger lesions can cause symptoms and are studied radiologically (Figs. 92 and 93). Adenomas are considered to be potentially premalignant lesions, and therefore their identification assumes definite importance.

There is no general agreement among pathologists concerning the relationship between renal adenoma and adenocarcinoma. Some believe that adenomas are generally not premalignant lesions. Some regard certain adenomas as premalignant lesions with a tendency to metastasize when they reach a certain size. Others believe that all adenomas are potentially malignant and do not find that histologic appearance or even size enables a clear distinction to be made. Bennington wrote that adenomas are in reality small renal carcinomas which usually metastasize after reaching a particular size: "Smaller tumors producing metastases and large tumors failing to metastasize are regarded as examples of extremes in the normal statistical distribution of biological phenomena."

An adenoma and a well-differentiated adenocarcinoma cannot be differentiated histologically. The only evidence that points to malignancy is the behavior of the tumor: Has it metastasized outside of the kidney, extended into venous structures, invaded the capsule? Many pathologists arbitrarily classify lesions less than 3 cm in size as benign adenomas and those over 3 cm as adenocarcinomas. However, the final decision as to whether a particular lesion is a benign or a malignant neoplasm depends ultimately on a long follow-up for evidence of recurrent disease.

HEMANGIOMA

Hemangioma is an exceedingly rare benign tumor of the kidney. Bell observed only one in 30,000 autopsies. Waller, Throckmorton and Barbosa collected 78 cases from the world literature up to 1955.

These tumors may involve the cortex, medulla or the subepithelial zone of the pelvis. They are generally venous in composition but may be arterial or mixed. They may be capillary but are generally of the cavernous type. Most are small, and many may not be recognized until postnephrectomy examination of the specimen. The main sign is hematuria. It is usually those lesions located in juxtaposition to the pelvis or renal sinus and particularly the papillary tumors that, following erosion of the urinary epithelium, cause bleeding.

Roentgen examination until recently has had only limited value in the demonstration of these growths. Pyelography may reveal a localized defect or deformity of the renal pelvis or calyx. However, in 1964 Andersen and Rasmussen diagnosed a renal hemangioma preoperatively by selective renal angiography. The use of renal angiography now permits recognition of these rare benign growths. In the past two years we have detected and studied two hemangiomas by renal angiography (Figs. 94 and 95). Both were in young patients with a history of intermittent hematuria. The capillary, cavernous and venous types differ in their angiographic appearance. The capillary form consists of a localized collection of small tightly bunched, coiled and tortuous vessels which produce a dense stain in the nephrogram phase (Fig. 95). The venous hemangioma consists of many dilated blood spaces in which the contrast medium collects in an uneven spotty manner (Fig. 94).

ANGIOMYOLIPOMA (HAMARTOMA)

Angiomyolipomas are composed of tissues of mixed mesenchymal origin. The tumors are made up of blood vessels, smooth muscle and fatty tissue. Depending on which tissues predominate, they may sometimes be classified as angiomyomas or myolipomas. Benign mesenchymoma is another pathologic term used to describe this entity.

Three apparently distinct patterns have been noted associated with angiomyolipoma. The first is the incidental discovery of these tumors at postmortem examination. In this instance, the tumors may be single or multiple, are usually quite small (less than 1 cm in size) and are not associated with clinical symptomatology. The second pattern is the association of hamartomas with tuberous sclerosis, and the third is the finding of single large angiomyolipomas which are symptomatic and usually are seen in women in the fifth and sixth decades. The latter two instances have clinical importance and are demonstrated in Figures 96 and 97.

LIPOMA

Lipomas are comparatively rare tumors of the kidney, usually encountered at autopsy as small, single tumors in the renal cortex. Occasionally they are multiple and found in the subcapsular area of the kidney. On occasion, lipomas may grow large enough in size to cause symptoms (usually flank pain) or radiologic signs (see Fig. 97–1). Those lesions causing symptoms are usually over 3 cm in size and lesions up to 10 cm in diameter have been recorded.

Radiologically these lesions are indistinguishable from other parenchymal tumors of the kidney except for the fat content of the tumor which (if the lesion is large enough) will show as a lucent shadow on the scout film of the abdomen (Fig. 97–1, *A*). In general, however, these tumors cannot be distinguished from more serious tumors and surgery with histologic identification is necessary for diagnosis (Fig. 97–1).

BIBLIOGRAPHY

Andersen, J. B., and Rasmussen, R.: Renal haemangioma diagnosed preoperatively by selective renal angiography, Acta radiol. (diag.) 2:201, 1964.

Bell, E. T.: Classification of renal tumors, with observations of the frequency of the various types, J. Urol. 29:238, 1938.

Bennington, J. L., and Kradjian, R. M.: *Renal Carcinoma* (Philadelphia: W. B. Saunders Company, 1967).

Lucké, B., and Schlumberger, H. G.: "Tumors of the Kidney, Renal Pelvis and Ureter;" Sec. VIII, Fasc. 30 of Armed Forces Institute of Pathology *Atlas of Tumor Pathology* (Washington, D.C.: 1957).

Thackry, A. C.: Benign Epithelial Tumours. In Riches, E. (ed.): *Tumours of the Kidney and Ureter* (Baltimore: Williams & Wilkins Company, 1964).

Waller, J. L.; Throckmorton, M. A., and Barbosa, E.: Renal hemangioma, J. Urol. 24: 86, 1955.

Figure 92.—Renal cortical adenoma.

A, selective right renal arteriogram, arterial phase, anteroposterior exposure: Demonstrating minimal hypervascularity and splaying and irregularity of arteries in the cortical zone between the middle and lower poles of the kidney (**arrows**).

B, same study, nephrogram phase: Showing the nephrogram in the area of the small cortical mass to be uneven and irregular. There is also loss of the normal cortical rim in this region (**arrow**).

A 44-year-old physician entered the hospital for examination after finding a neck mass during shaving. Intravenous urography revealed a small mass in the outer aspect of the right kidney. A right nephrectomy was performed and a 3 cm cortical adenoma was identified. He subsequently died of widespread metastatic disease from a primary carcinoma of the lung.

Comment: Angiographically this lesion must be considered malignant and is indistinguishable from a small renal carcinoma. Pathologically the lesion might be considered benign by some pathologists and malignant or premalignant by others. Most pathologists believe that the gross size determines whether a particular lesion should be classified as benign or malignant, using 3 cm diameter as the critical measurement.* Histologically, cortical adenoma cannot be differentiated from adenocarcinoma unless invasion of capsule, veins or other structures can be detected.

---

* Bell, E. T.: *Renal Disease* (5th ed.; Philadelphia: Lea & Febiger, 1947), p. 422.

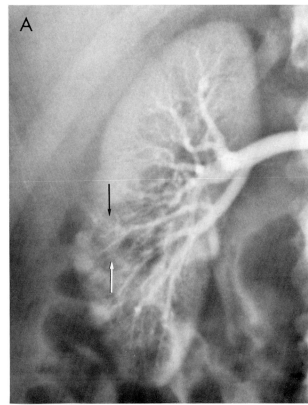

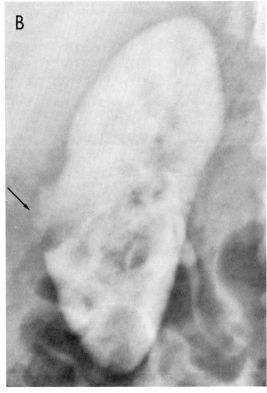

Figure 92 · Renal Cortical Adenoma / 281

Figure 93.—Papillary adenoma (adenocarcinoma).

A, nephrotomogram, anteroposterior projection: Revealing a centrally located intrarenal mass (**arrows**).

B, selective right renal arteriogram, early phase, anteroposterior view: Delineating some stretching of vessels around a mass in the midpole of the kidney (**x**) but no abnormal vessels.

C, same study, nephrogram phase: Showing the mass well outlined by a dense thickened wall (**arrows**). Its center is lucent.

A middle-aged man was hospitalized after an episode of hematuria. An intravenous urogram suggested a mass in the midportion of the right kidney. A right nephrectomy was performed and a well-encapsulated lesion 4 cm in diameter was found. The histologic diagnosis was papillary adenoma, but because it measured more than 3 cm it could also be considered to be an adenocarcinoma. The benignancy or malignancy of these lesions is difficult to evaluate, and their future course (whether they metastasize or not) determines their true nature.

Figure 93, courtesy of Dr. Joshua A. Becker, State University of New York, Downstate Medical Center, Brooklyn, New York.

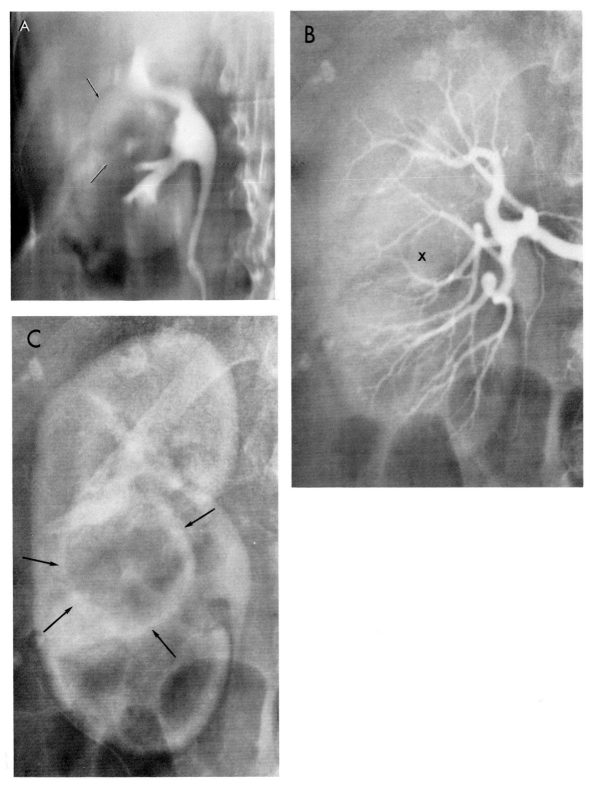

Figure 93 · Papillary Adenoma (Adenocarcinoma) / 283

Figure 94.—Venous hemangioma.

A, intravenous urogram, anteroposterior projection: Showing normal appearance of the right kidney. The axis of the left calyceal system appears to be rotated and the lower calyces are poorly filled. The lower lateral margin of the left kidney is poorly defined.

B, retrograde aortogram, aortic phase, anteroposterior exposure: Revealing a single right renal artery. The left kidney has two renal arteries, one to the upper half (**X**) and one to the lower half (**Y**). There is no evidence of neoplastic vasculature in the arterial phase.

C, same study, nephrogram phase: Clearly demonstrating a circumscribed mass occupying the lower pole of the left kidney and causing a distinct bulge of the lateral contour of the kidney. The mass is unevenly radiolucent. Vessels seen at the lower pole of the left kidney are intestinal vessels that are still opacified.

(*Continued* on p. 286.)

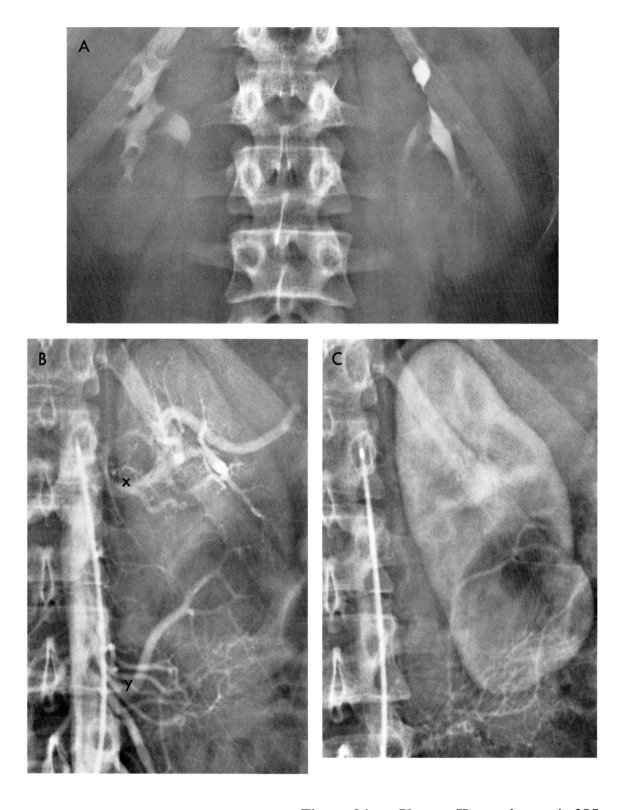

Figure 94 · Venous Hemangioma / 285

Figure 94 (cont).—Venous hemangioma.

D, selective angiogram of left inferior renal artery, arterial phase, anteroposterior view: Delineating a few small tortuous and dilated vessels in the midportion of the kidney (**arrows**). Note stretching of vessels in the lower pole.

E, same study, nephrogram phase: Revealing small opaque collections (**x**) within a largely radiolucent mass. One prominent vein (**arrow**) lies just lateral to the renal contour.

A man of 25 was hospitalized because of gross hematuria. His symptoms first appeared at age 7 and recurred about every one or two years, lasting one or two days. After left nephrectomy, pathologic examination revealed the medulla of the lower pole to be replaced by small cystic structures measuring up to 3 cm in greatest diameter. The cysts were filled with dark blood. The cortex was not involved. Histologic diagnosis was hemangioma.

Comment: This is an example of a large venous hemangioma not well seen on the intravenous urogram. The selective renal angiogram (**D** and **E**) shows the entire lower pole of the kidney to be occupied by a large (6 $\times$ 8.5 cm), unevenly radiolucent mass within which are focal collections of contrast medium (**E, x**). Cystlike venous lakes comprise the main mass of the hemangioma. The large vein (**E, arrow**) on the surface of the kidney communicated with the internal hemangioma. This venous hemangioma, like the capillary or cavernous variety, has a somewhat characteristic angiographic appearance, permitting a possible preoperative diagnosis. However, the possibility of a cystic malignancy could not be excluded on the basis of the angiogram in this case.

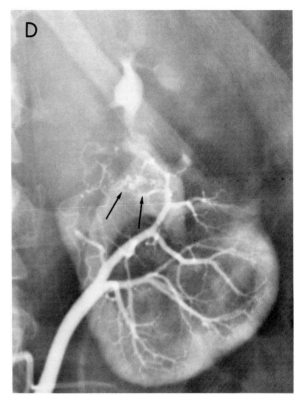

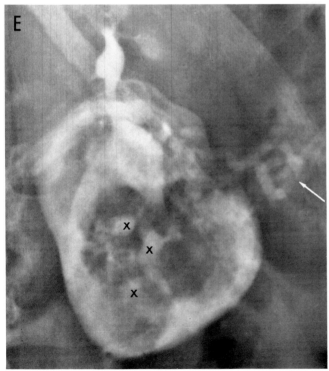

Figure 94 · Venous Hemangioma / 287

Figure 95.—Cavernous hemangioma of the kidney.

A, intravenous urogram, anteroposterior view: Revealing no abnormalities in the collecting system of the right kidney, which seems grossly normal in size and outline. The small density above the upper pole calyx was proved to be outside the kidney.

B, selective right renal arteriogram, arterial phase, anteroposterior view: Showing the main renal artery to be of normal size. A small localized collection of intensely opacified tortuous vessels is seen in the midportion of the upper pole (**arrow**), with some hypertrophy of the arterial branch feeding these vessels, which border on the renal sinus. There is no mass effect, displacement of vessels or arteriovenous shunting.

C, same study, nephrogram phase: Showing the collection of vessels in the upper pole to better advantage than in **B.** The vessels have a tortuous, coiled appearance but are regular and provide an intense stain (**arrow**).

D, same study after 8 μg of epinephrine: Intensifying the image of the vascular lesion because the rest of the renal vessels are constricted and thus not filled. Note the excellent delineation of the adrenal gland (**arrow**), which is not uncommon when epinephrine is used. (Presumably the adrenal vessels are not as sensitive to epinephrine as are renal vessels, so that more perfusion of contrast medium takes place through them.)

Two years before this study, after a dose of Butazolidin, this woman of 40 had massive gross hematuria and later had two similar episodes. A right heminephrectomy revealed a small cavernous hemangioma.

Comment: The diagnosis of hemangioma of the kidney can be suggested on the basis of its angiographic appearance. A small vascular malignancy would be difficult to differentiate, however. This case is a good example of the capillary or cavernous type of hemangioma. It also reveals the nonspecificity of the epinephrine test in angiography and shows that abnormal vessels of a hemangioma will also not respond to epinephrine.

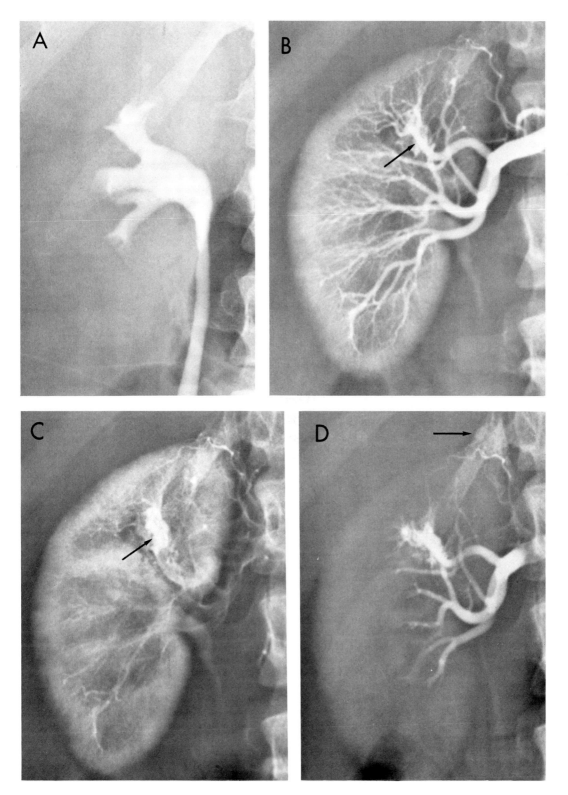

Figure 95 · Cavernous Hemangioma / 289

Figure 96.—Multiple hamartomas (angiomyolipomas) of the kidney in a patient with tuberous sclerosis.

A, intravenous urogram (1962), anteroposterior exposure: Showing large kidneys. The unusual configuration of the calyces suggests multiple masses in both kidneys and is consistent with the calyceal pattern seen in angiomyolipomas.

B, intravenous urogram (1967), anteroposterior projection: Revealing the large left kidney exhibiting the same calyceal deformities that had been present in 1962. (The right kidney had been surgically removed.)

C, retrograde aortogram (1967), anteroposterior projection: Delineating three large renal arteries (**arrows**) supplying the huge left kidney. Extensive irregular vascularity fills the kidney. The superior mesenteric artery (**a**) courses to the right.

(*Continued* on p. 292.)

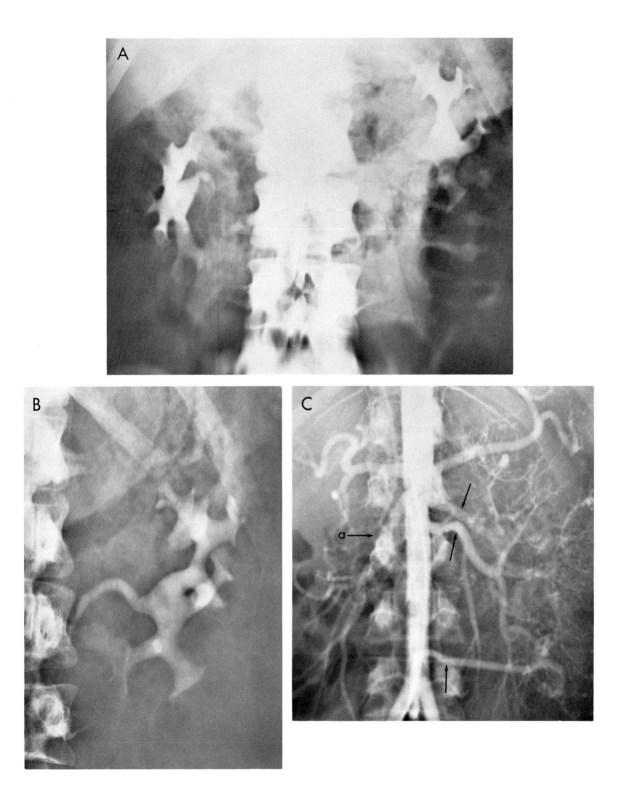

Figure 96 · Angiomyolipomas & Tuberous Sclerosis / 291

Figure 96 (cont.).—Multiple hamartomas (angiomyolipomas) of the kidney in a patient with tuberous sclerosis.

D, selective left renal arteriogram, arterial phase, anteroposterior view: With catheterization of the left middle renal artery demonstrating a bizarre arterial pattern of hypervascularity. The interlobar branches are large and show varying degrees of displacement. The smaller interlobular branches are tortuous, irregular and circinoid, and numerous small berrylike aneurysms are present throughout the vascular network. Despite the great vascularity there is no evidence of arteriovenous shunting.

E, same study, nephrogram phase: Demonstrating a diffuse spotty angiomatous pattern throughout this huge kidney.

A woman of 31, from South America, was hospitalized in August, 1967, because of left flank pain and a palpable mass. In 1962, she had had a right nephrectomy for what was said to be a malignant mesenchymoma. Histologic sections of the right kidney were reviewed in 1967 by an outstanding tumor pathologist, who diagnosed angiomyolipoma. Physical examination in 1967 revealed classic stigmas of tuberous sclerosis.

Comment: From 50–80% of patients with tuberous sclerosis have multiple hamartomas of the kidneys, and 50% of hamartomas are found in patients with tuberous sclerosis. Radiographic features in these cases are striking and diagnostic. The urographic pattern of enlarged kidneys with evidence of multiple renal masses resembles that of polycystic kidneys, but angiographic findings are quite distinctive of multiple hamartomas. The abnormal-appearing vessels are unusually circinoid and serpiginous, with outpouchings resembling small aneurysms (see also Fig. 97). There is puddling of contrast medium in these unusual vessels and the nephrogram phase shows an unusual but distinctive irregular pattern due to the various tissues making up these mixed tumors.*

---

* Viamonte, M., Jr.; Ravel, R.; Politano, V., and Bridges, B.: Angiographic findings in a patient with tuberous sclerosis, Am. J. Roentgenol. 98:723, 1966.

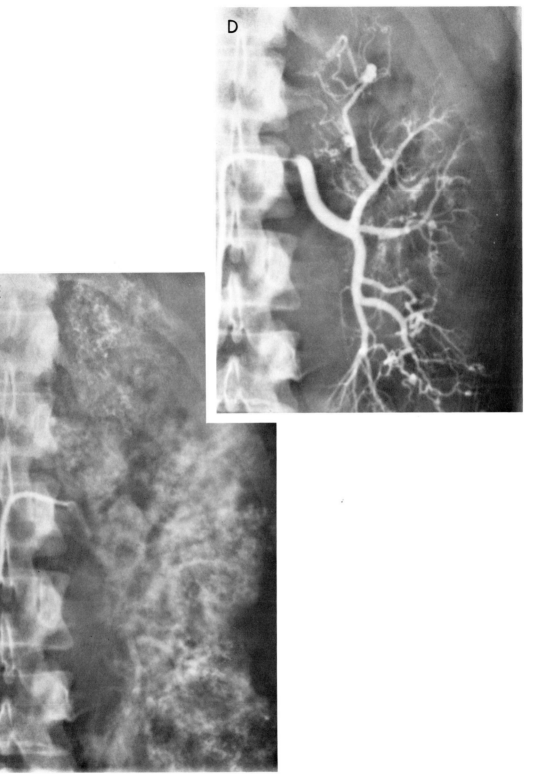

Figure 96 · Angiomyolipomas & Tuberous Sclerosis / 293

Figure 97.—Angiomyolipoma (hamartoma) of the kidney.

A, selective right renal arteriogram, anteroposterior exposure: Revealing hypertrophy of a branch of the renal artery supplying a vascular tumor originating at the lower pole of the kidney (**a**). Extremely tortuous, circinoid tumor vessels are present (**b**). A capsular artery is also supplying the tumor (**c**).

B, inferior venacavogram, anteroposterior view: Showing the inferior vena cava displaced to the midline by a large right-sided mass. There is poor function of the right kidney. Numerous radiolucent collections within the soft tissue mass (**arrows**) represent fat collections in the tumor.

A woman of 57 had a right-sided abdominal mass. Intravenous urography revealed a poorly functioning right kidney with a large mass at the lower pole which appeared to be partly radiolucent (see **B**). A right nephrectomy was performed for angiomyolipoma.

Comment: Angiomyolipomas also occur in patients without tuberous sclerosis. They are usually benign and single lesions and occur in women in the fifth and sixth decades.* (With tuberous sclerosis the lesions are usually multiple and bilateral; Fig. 96.) Because of the large amount of fatty tissue in these tumors a lucent mass may be seen in the urogram, which should suggest the correct diagnosis. The vascularity of most angiomyolipomas gives a rather distinctive angiographic pattern, the most striking feature being extreme tortuosity of the vessels with stasis and many small focal dilatations having the appearance of numerous berrylike aneurysms (see also Fig. 83).

---

* Love, L., and Frank, S. J.: Angiographic features of angiomyolipoma of kidney, Am. J. Roentgenol. 95:406, 1965.

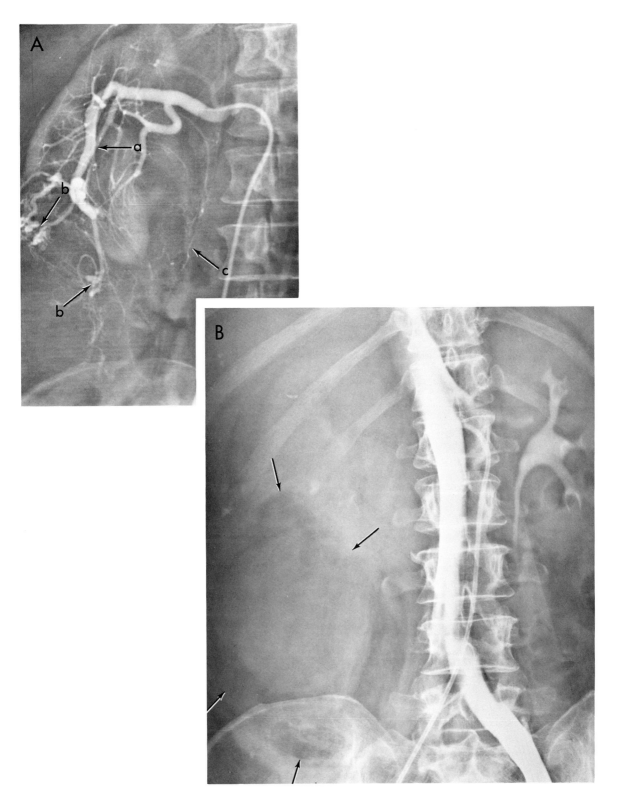

Figure 97 · Angiomyolipoma / 295

Figure 97–1.—Lipoma of the kidney.

A, scout film for intravenous urogram, anteroposterior projection: Showing the contour of the right kidney. Note area of lucency in midportion of the kidney (**arrows**).

B, intravenous urogram, anteroposterior projection: Revealing a mass in the midportion of the right kidney with a pressure deformity on the upper pole calyx and renal pelvis. Note that the mass has a lucent appearance corresponding to the area of lucency noted on the plain film, *A*.

C, selective right renal anteriogram, anteroposterior projection: Demonstrating displacement of the intrarenal branches about the mass. A few small abnormal-appearing vessels are seen associated with the tumor (**arrows**).

D, surgical specimen: Revealing a well circumscribed lipoma in the midportion of the kidney.

The patient was a 54-year-old female who had been previously treated for tuberculosis. A routine intravenous urogram demonstrated a right renal mass. A right nephrectomy was performed. Microscopic examination revealed a typical lipoma with vacuolated fat cells. Scattered throughout the lipoma were small, feeding arteries.

Comment: In this case, the diagnosis of a fat-containing tumor could be suggested by the observation of the relative lucency of the intrarenal mass on the scout film. However, the angiogram revealed some abnormal-appearing vessels associated with the mass so that a malignant tumor could not be excluded until nephrectomy and histologic examination were performed. Even the epinephrine test, which was performed in this case, indicated abnormal vasculature so that the benign nature of the lesion could not be suspected preoperatively.

Lipomas are rare neoplasms of the kidney. In most instances, they are discovered incidentally at autopsy, but occasionally reach large enough size to be studied clinically, as in this case.

The observation that the mass was lucent on the scout film should suggest a lipomatous element to the lesion. Other lesions that contain fat include liposarcomas and mixed mesenchymal tumors, including angiomyolipomas (both benign and malignant), so that exploratory surgery and histologic identification are necessary in the evaluation of these fat-containing tumors.

Figure 97–1, courtesy of Schield, P. N.: Epinephrine effect in the vascular pattern of a renal lipoma, Radiology 59:657, 1970.

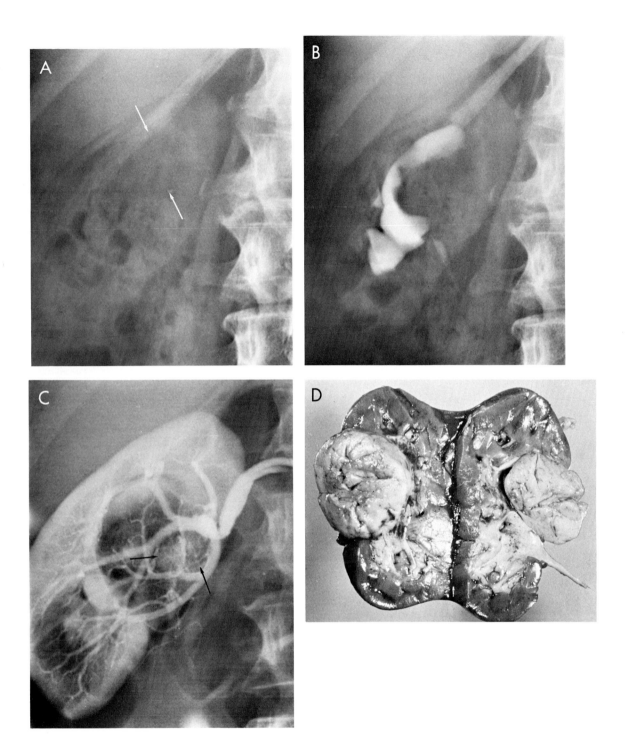

Figure 97–1 · Lipoma of the Kidney / 297

PART 6

Pseudotumors of the Renal Parenchyma

Characteristics of Renal Parenchyma Pseudotumors

PSEUDOTUMORS of the kidney are a heterogeneous collection of lesions which on conventional urography closely simulate the appearance of true renal neoplasms or cysts. Familiarity with these entities is essential if they are to be successfully differentiated from true tumors. These spurious renal masses form a spectrum of diverse entities, including congenital lobulations (Figs. 98 and 99), congenital anomalies of the kidney including prominent renal column (Fig. 100), localized hydronephrosis (Figs. 102 and 103), focal hyperplasia secondary to chronic pyelonephritis, arteriovenous malformation (Fig. 107), focal fibrolipomatosis (Fig. 101), hematoma (Fig. 108), inflammatory granuloma (Fig. 104), abscess (Fig. 105), xanthogranulomatous pyelonephritis (Fig. 106) and fresh infarct.

The true nature of most of these pseudotumors can be recognized by the use of such specialized methods as nephrotomography and renal angiography. It is important, therefore, that patients with urographic evidence suggesting a renal tumor be given the benefit of a complete radiologic study. Failure to do so may well result in unnecessary renal exploration and even loss of a normal kidney.

Figure 98.—Congenital lobulation.

Nephrotomogram, anteroposterior exposure: Revealing lobulation of the outer aspect of the right kidney (**arrow**). Incidentally, this nephrotomogram also demonstrates very well a slight increase in the amount of fat in the left renal sinus.

Comment: Congenital lobulation is a rather common anatomic variant in the renal contour. It most often involves the midlateral margin of the kidney but may be observed in the polar regions as well as the renal hilus. It may mimic a renal mass and at times may suggest localized cortical atrophy secondary to focal pyelonephritis or renal infarction.* Nephrotomography is very helpful in differentiating congenital lobulations from serious renal pathology.

---

* Cooperman, L. R., and Lowman, R. M.: Fetal lobulation of the kidneys, Am. J. Roentgenol. 92:273, 1964.

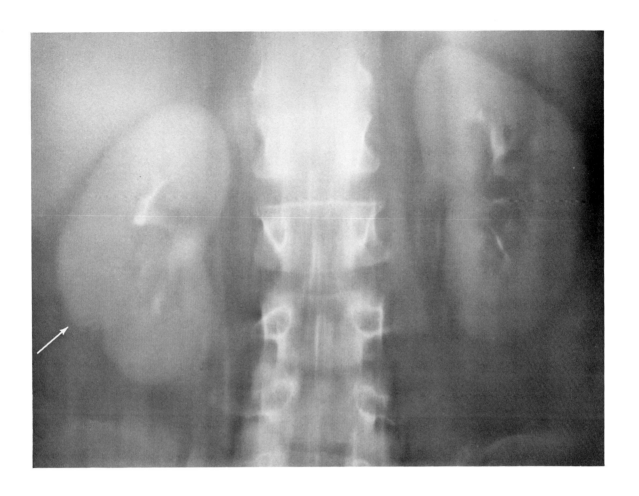

Figure 98 · Congenital Lobulation / 303

Figure 99.—Cortical lobulation.

A, intravenous urogram, anteroposterior projection: Revealing a bulbous lower pole of the right kidney (**arrows**) with a suggestion of distortion of the lower pole calyx.

B, nephrotomogram: Showing the lower pole of the kidney to be bulbous but apparently containing normal renal parenchyma, since the nephrogram in this area is normal with no evidence of lucency to suggest a cyst or increased density to suggest a tumor.

C, selective right renal arteriogram, arterial phase, anteroposterior view: Demonstrating no abnormal vascularity. There is no displacement of vessels or abnormality in their perfusion.

D, same study, nephrogram phase: Presenting a normal nephrogram. The bulbous lower pole is well demonstrated. The lucencies over the lower pole represent gas in the overlying bowel.

The patient was a 45-year-old woman who was hospitalized for investigation of hypertension.

Comment: Occasionally congenital lobulation of the renal cortex is so pronounced that nephrotomography or renal arteriography or both are necessary to rule out tumor, as in this case.

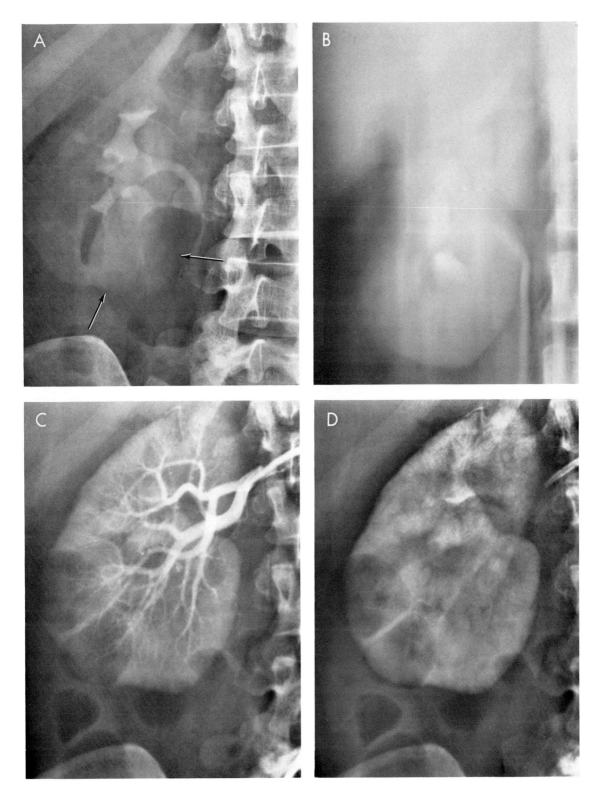

Figure 99 · Cortical Lobulation / 305

Figure 100.—Pseudotumor caused by normal renal cortical tissue projecting into the renal sinus (renal column).

A, intravenous urogram, anteroposterior projection: Revealing a suggestion of a mass between the upper and middle pole calyces of the right kidney (**x**).

(*Continued* on p. 308.)

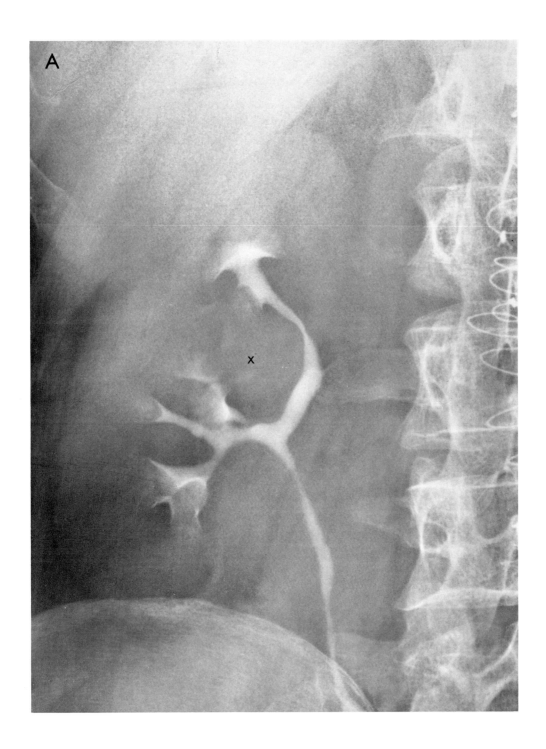

Figure 100 · Renal Column / 307

Figure 100 (cont.).—Pseudotumor caused by normal renal cortical tissue projecting into the renal sinus (renal column).

B, right selective renal arteriogram, arterial phase, anteroposterior view: Delineating apparently normal intrarenal vasculature and no tumor vessels. Note stretching of major renal artery branches around the area of the apparent mass.

C, same study, nephrogram phase: Demonstrating a well-defined stain in the area of the apparent mass (**a**). The density of the "mass" is the same as that of the renal cortex (**b**).

A man of 62 had symptoms of prostatism. Because of the possibility of a renal neoplasm, the right kidney was explored. It was normal externally, but because of the mistaken belief that the lesion represented a neoplasm, nephrectomy was performed. Pathologic examination revealed a normal kidney. The area of suspected abnormality represented invagination of cortical tissue toward the renal sinus impinging on the collecting system in this area.

Comment: This case is characteristic of the pseudotumor caused by the so-called renal column.* Knowledge of this anatomic variation is extremely important if the circumstances of this case are not to be duplicated. Five similar cases have been sent us that demonstrated the same findings. These pseudotumors almost always occur between the middle and upper pole calyces and are usually well marginated medially because they are surrounded by renal sinus fat. Angiographically there is stretching of the main intrarenal branches around these pseudotumors with blood supply coming from short direct secondary branches. No abnormal vessels are present, and the density of the nephrogram in the pseudotumor is similar to that of cortical tissue in the periphery of the kidney.

Figure 100, courtesy of Dr. Theodore Robinson, State University of New York, Downstate Medical Center, Brooklyn, New York.

---

* King, M. C.; Friedenberg, R. M., and Tena, L. B.: Normal renal parenchyma simulating tumor, Radiology 91:217, 1968.

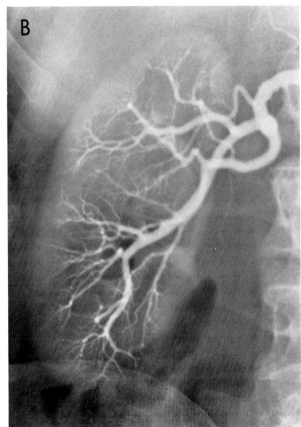

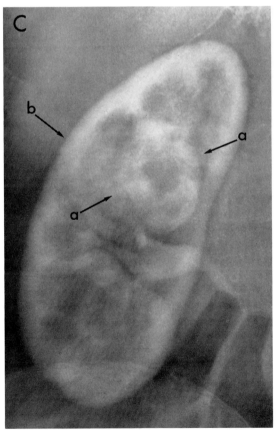

Figure 100 · Renal Column / 309

Figure 101.—Pseudotumor caused by localized renal sinus lipomatosis.

A, intravenous urogram, anteroposterior projection: Showing a pressure deformity involving the left renal pelvis and middle pole calyces (**arrows**).

B, nephrotomogram, anteroposterior exposure: Showing the peripelvic mass to be lucent but not round and symmetrical (**arrows**). Smaller lucencies around the upper pole calyces (**x**) represent normal renal sinus fat.

A man of 63 entered the hospital because of symptoms of prostatism. On exploration the kidney seemed normal externally. Needle aspiration of the peripelvic area yielded no fluid or abnormal collections. The diagnosis was then presumed to be a large collection of renal sinus lipomatosis.

Comment: Because of the lucency of this mass on nephrotomography it was thought that the lesion was not a solid tumor but might be either a peripelvic cyst or fibrolipomatosis. Often the two cannot be differentiated radiographically (including angiography). Nevertheless the surgeon decided on exploration, and failure to obtain cyst fluid suggested that the diagnosis was lipomatosis. Such a kidney would no longer be explored, since further radiologic experience with this type of lesion has been accumulated.

Renal sinus lipomatosis is the deposition of excessive amounts of fat in the renal sinus. Innocuous in its effect on the patient, the condition assumes major clinical importance by producing pelvocalyceal deformities suggestive of renal tumors or cysts. In most instances, lipomatosis presents a characteristic nephrotomographic appearance and is readily differentiated from true renal masses.*

---

* Faegenburg, D.; Bosniak, M. A., and Evans, J. A.: Renal sinus lipomatosis: Its demonstration by nephrotomography, Radiology 83:987, 1964.

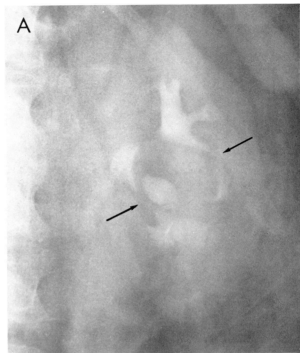

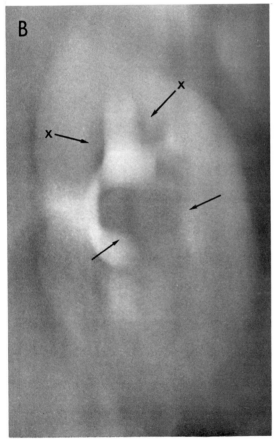

Figure 101 · Localized Lipomatosis / 311

Figure 102.—Pseudotumor due to localized hydronephrosis.

A, intravenous urogram, anteroposterior projection: Revealing a large mass occupying the lower half of the right kidney (**arrows**) and causing ureterectasis and caliectasis of the collecting system visualized.

(*Continued* on p. 314.)

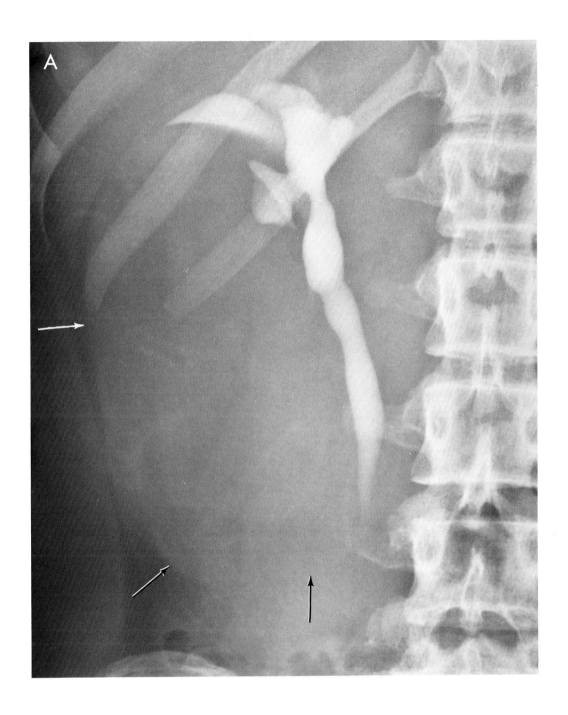

Figure 102 · Localized Hydronephrosis / 313

Figure 102 (cont.).—Pseudotumor due to localized hydronephrosis.

B, aortogram, anteroposterior exposure: Indicating that the main renal artery is normal as well as the intrarenal branches in the upper portion of the kidney. Arteries in the middle and lower portions of the kidney are atrophic, stretched and attenuated, and their terminal branching is poorly demonstrated.

C, selective right renal arteriogram, late phase: Showing a normal nephrogram in the upper portion of the kidney. Vessels in the lower portion of the kidney stretch around a large lucent mass. Note, however, that the mass has a thickened wall—the rim sign of hydronephrosis (**arrows**).

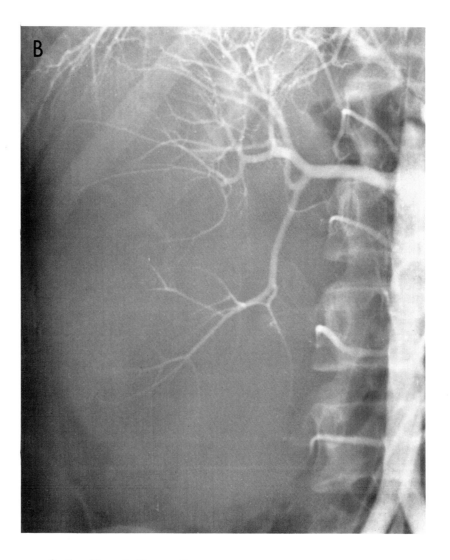

A 16-year-old girl was hospitalized because of a right-sided abdominal mass, fever and pain. Surgery revealed a large infected hydronephrotic sac replacing the lower two-thirds of the kidney, and nephrectomy was performed. A congenital stricture in a bifid renal pelvis was found.

Comment: Hydronephrosis, when localized to one portion of the kidney, may be very difficult to differentiate from a renal neoplasm. The angiographic findings in the hydronephrotic segment can resemble those of a hypovascular neoplasm. However, if the possibility of a duplicated collecting system is considered, diagnosis is possible (see Bosniak *et al.* below).

Figure 102, courtesy of Bosniak, M. A.; Scheff, S., and Kaufman, S.: Localized hydronephrosis masquerading as renal neoplasm, J. Urol. 99:241, 1968.

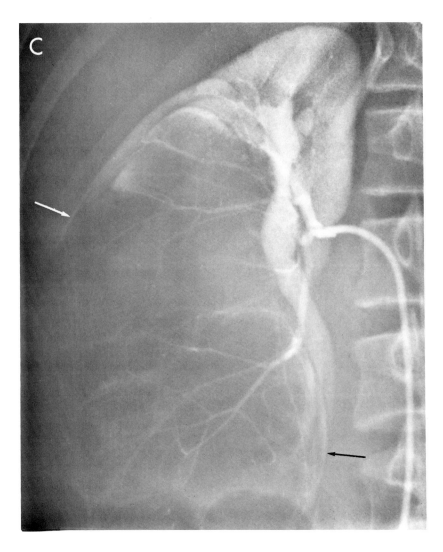

Figure 102 · Localized Hydronephrosis / 315

Figure 103.—Pseudotumor due to hydronephrosis of a duplicated collecting system.

A, intravenous urogram, anteroposterior projection: In which the right kidney appears to be displaced laterally and slightly downward by a large mass above and medial to the kidney.

B, same study, delayed film: Revealing a collection of contrast medium in the upper pole of the kidney (**arrows**) indicating that the pseudotumor represents localized hydronephrosis of the upper portion of a duplicated collecting system.

Two months before this examination a 15-year-old boy injured his right side while playing basketball. That night he had gross hematuria. A right nephrectomy was performed after an attempt at partial nephrectomy was unsuccessful. The specimen revealed a congenital anomaly of the right kidney

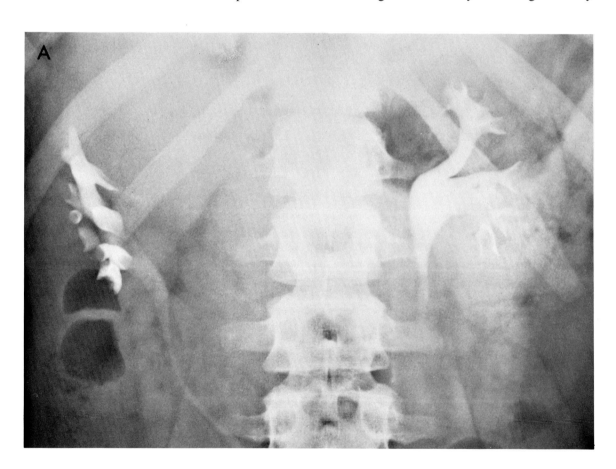

with a duplicated collecting system. There were chronic hydronephrosis and pyelonephritis of the upper portion.

Comment: The number and distribution of the calyces of the lower component of the duplicated system on the right could be mistaken for a complete kidney. It is this deceptive appearance that causes the hydronephrotic upper system to simulate an intrarenal tumor or an extrarenal mass displacing the kidney. However, on the delayed film the hydronephrotic portion of the kidney opacifies, clarifying the diagnosis.

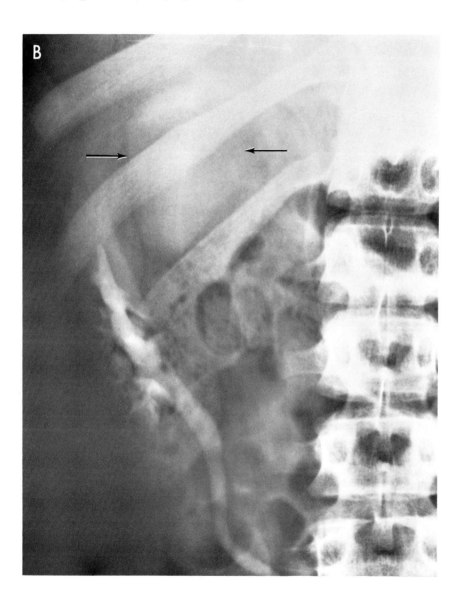

Figure 103 · Localized Hydronephrosis / 317

Figure 104.—Pseudotumor due to tuberculomas.

A, intravenous urogram, anteroposterior projection: Revealing stippled calcific densities in the renal cortex just above and lateral to the upper pole calyx (**arrow**), which is apparently amputated. There is increased distance between the upper pole calyx and the upper margin of the kidney (**a**). A similar appearance is seen at the lower pole (**b**), suggesting masses in both areas.

(*Continued* on p. 320.)

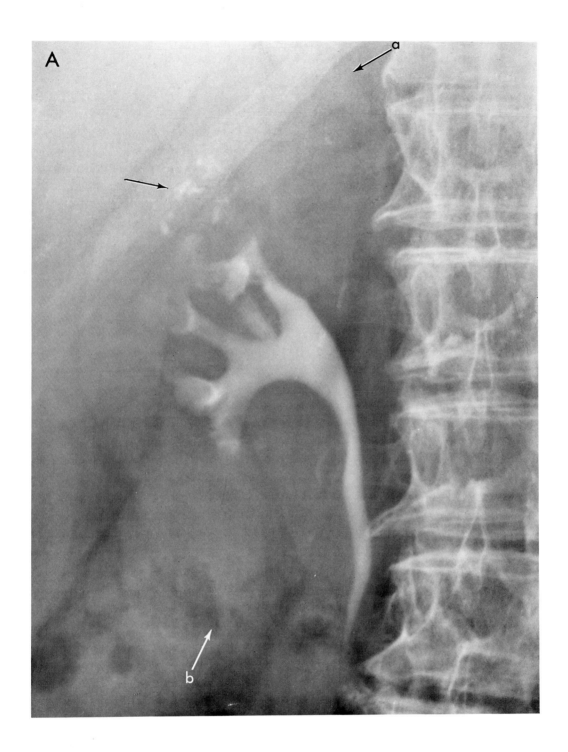

Figure 104 · Tuberculomas / 319

Figure 104 (cont.).—Pseudotumor due to tuberculomas.

B, selective right renal arteriogram, arterial phase, anteroposterior exposure: Showing the main renal artery to be narrowed at its origin (**arrow**). Diminished vascularity is evident in the upper and lower poles. No abnormal vessels are seen, but the vessels delineated are attenuated.

C, same study, nephrogram phase: Revealing relatively lucent upper and lower pole masses with thick walls (**arrows**). Only the central portion of the kidney has a normal nephrogram.

A man of 67 was hospitalized because of "colitis." A routine chest radiograph revealed a mass in the left upper lobe. A percutaneous needle biopsy specimen was reported to show "metastatic adenocarcinoma suggestive of renal origin." A right nephrectomy was performed. Numerous caseous tuberculous granulomas were present in both poles of the kidney. The largest at the upper pole measured 5.2 cm in diameter and at the lower pole, 3 cm in diameter. The wall of the larger upper pole granuloma contained deposits of calcium.

Comment: Angiographically, tuberculous granulomas can be quite difficult to distinguish from hypovascular necrotic renal neoplasm. Usually, urographic findings distinguish these entities. However, when the lesion is mainly parenchymal in origin differentiation becomes more difficult.* In this case the amputation of the calyx, stippled calcification and multiplicity of the lesions are a clue to the infectious origin of these masses, but generally the diagnosis cannot be made in lesions of the type depicted in this case without a strong clinical history indicating tuberculosis.

Figure 104, courtesy of Drs. Lawrence H. Caplan and Benjamin Harrow, Miami, Fla.

---

* Bjorn-Hansen, R., and Aakhus, T.: Angiography in renal tuberculosis, Acta radiol. (diag.) 11:167, 1971.

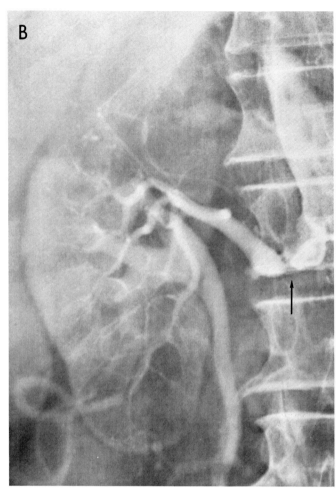

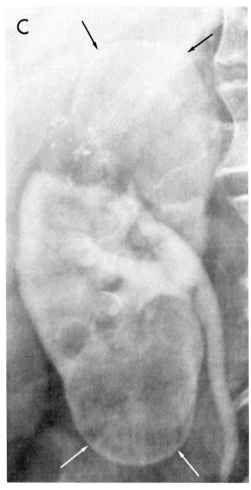

Figure 104 · Tuberculomas / 321

Figure 105.—Pseudotumor due to an intrarenal abscess.

    A, intravenous urogram, anteroposterior projection: Revealing a normal right kidney. In the left kidney there are poor filling and visualization of the middle and lower pole calyces, which appear to be slightly spread, suggesting the possibility of a mass in this area. Also, the renal margin is ill-defined in the lateral aspect of the kidney.

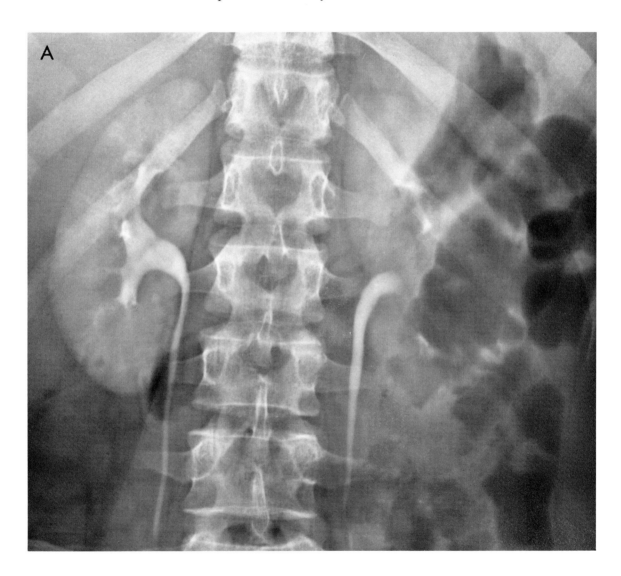

B, nephrotomogram, anteroposterior view: Suggesting a mass in the outer midpole of the left kidney with pressure on the collecting system (**x**). Note irregularity of the cortical margin (**arrow**).

(*Continued* on p. 324.)

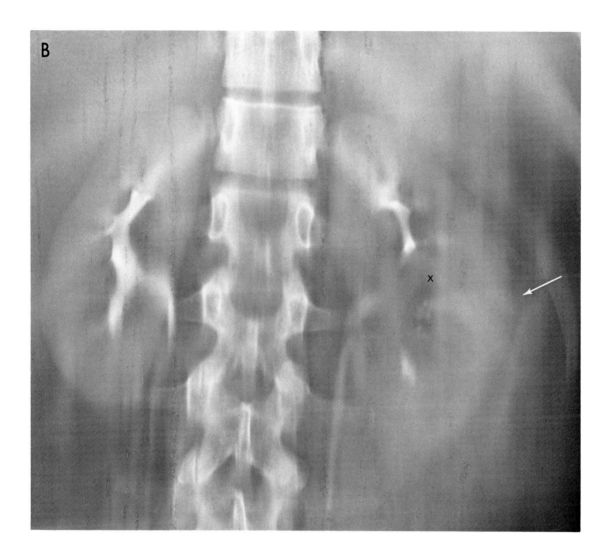

Figure 105 · Intrarenal Abscess / 323

Figure 105 (cont.).—Pseudotumor due to an intrarenal abscess.

C, selective left renal arteriogram, left posterior oblique projection: Showing evident stretching of vessels in the midportion of the kidney. Note the loss of nephrogram in the cortex (**arrows**) and irregular margin of the kidney in this area.

A 17-year-old girl complained of variable but persistent left flank pain accompanied by daily afternoon fever. Exploratory surgery revealed a large acute abscess on the anterior surface of the kidney cortex which was incised and drained.

Comment: The findings in this case are not specific for abscess but suggest a poorly defined mass in the renal cortex. The radiologic picture ruled out a simple benign cyst, so exploratory surgery was indicated.

An acute abscess may not present abnormal vasculature. Subacute and chronic abscesses are usually associated with some increased vascularity to the capsule and therefore cannot be distinguished radiologically from hypovascular malignancy (see Fig. 106).

Renal abscess can be a difficult condition to diagnose preoperatively.* In this case, the diagnosis of renal abscess was made because it was suspected clinically and the radiologic changes were consistent with the clinical impression.

---

* Evans, J. A., Meyers, M. A., and Bosniak, M. A.: Acute renal and perirenal infections, Seminars in Roentgenol. 6:274, 1971.

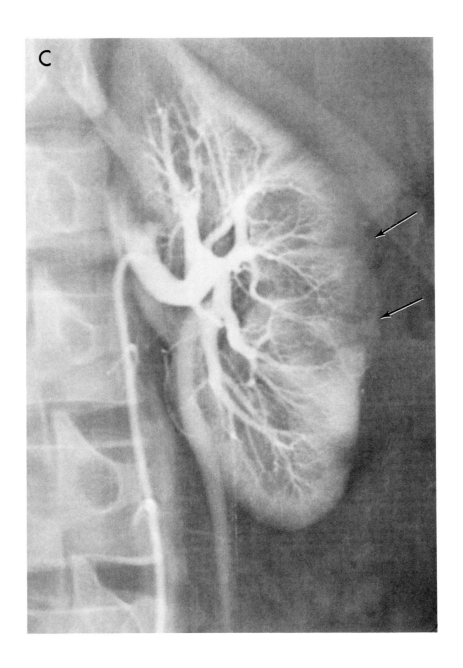

Figure 105 · Intrarenal Abscess / 325

Figure 106.—Pseudotumor due to xanthogranulomatous pyelonephritis with perirenal extension.

A, right retrograde pyelogram, anteroposterior projection: Revealing a displaced, distorted and contracted collecting system of the right kidney. There is a large mass in the right flank but its margins are ill-defined.

B, selective right renal arteriogram, arterial phase, anteroposterior view: Showing distorted and displaced intrarenal branches. Intrarenally there is increased vascularity. Some abnormal-appearing vessels, which are perforating vessels from the kidney, extend into the perirenal space (**a**). There is also enlargement and medial displacement of renal pelvic and capsular arteries (**b**).

(*Continued* on p. 328.)

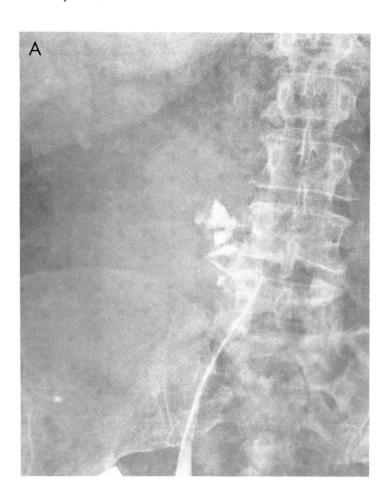

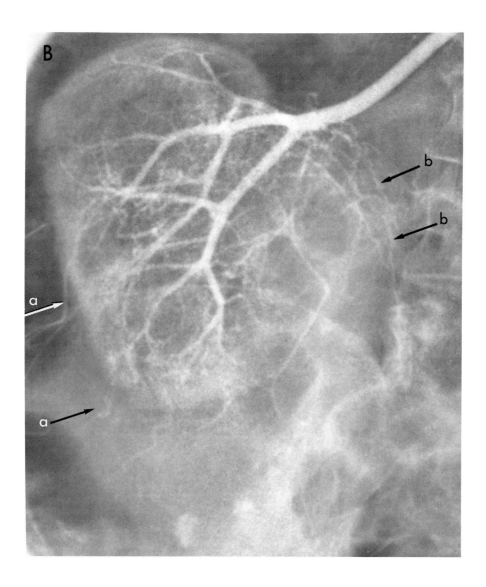

Figure 106 · Xanthogranulomatous Pyelonephritis / 327

Figure 106 (cont.).—Pseudotumor due to xanthogranulomatous pyelonephritis with perirenal extension.

C, same study, nephrogram phase: Showing an irregular, spotty nephrogram. The kidney margin is indistinct, particularly medially, and there is a contrast medium blush in the perirenal areas (**arrows**), indicating extension of the process into the perirenal space.

A woman of 56 had fever and a palpable right-sided abdominal mass. An intravenous urogram revealed no visualization of the right kidney but a large soft tissue mass in the right flank. Exploration disclosed the right kidney fixed within a large thick-walled mass of inflammatory tissue. Biopsy study revealed chronic inflammation and xanthogranulomatous pyelonephritis. When she eventually died of other causes, autopsy confirmed these findings.

Comment: Chronic renal and perirenal abscess and xanthogranulomatous pyelonephritis can be difficult to distinguish radiologically from renal malignancy. Mass effect and increased vascularity with abnormal-appearing vessels are seen in all of these conditions. Preoperative diagnosis of renal abscess (or xanthogranulomatous pyelonephritis) in many instances may not be possible unless there is a strong clinical history of renal infection (see Caplan *et al.* below).

Figure 106, courtesy of Caplan, L. H.; Siegelman, S. S., and Bosniak, M. A.: Angiography in inflammatory space-occupying lesions of the kidney, Radiology 88:14, 1967.

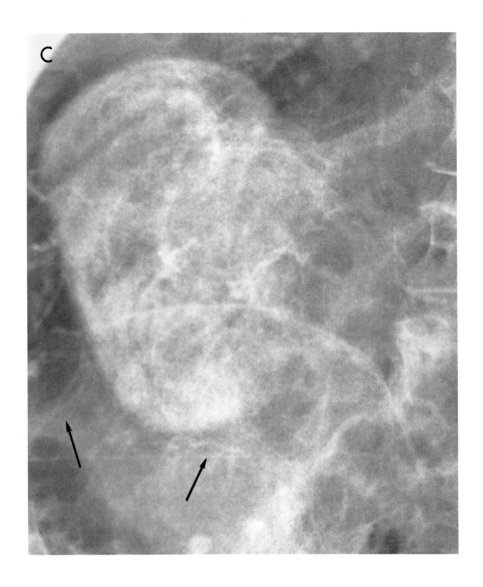

Figure 106 · Xanthogranulomatous Pyelonephritis / 329

Figure 107.—Pseudotumor due to a large arteriovenous malformation.

A, retrograde pyelogram, right kidney, anteroposterior view: Revealing a parapelvic mass compressing and distorting the renal pelvis with some obstruction of the lower pole calyx.

B, selective right renal arteriogram, early phase, anteroposterior projection: Showing immediate filling of a large aneurysmal sac. Vessels to the lower pole are stretched over other portions of the arteriovenous malformation that are not opacified at this time (see **C** and **D**). A large cyst is present in the upper pole, as reflected by thin attenuated vessels in this part of the kidney.

C, same study, 2 seconds after **B:** Showing further filling of the vascular malformation.

D, same study, 2 seconds after **C:** Demonstrating continued opacification of the large malformation. A large venous aneurysmal sac is responsible for the parapelvic mass originally noted in the urogram. Filling of the renal vein and inferior vena cava is also seen (**arrows**).

A woman of 33 had a urinary tract infection. An intravenous urogram revealed poor visualization of the kidneys bilaterally and a suggestion of a mass in the right kidney.

Comment: An arteriovenous malformation frequently may present as a pseudotumor. Only angiography will differentiate this lesion from a renal neoplasm. Some arteriovenous malformations are associated with hypertension due to the arteriovenous shunt or renal ischemia, or both. This was not present in this case.

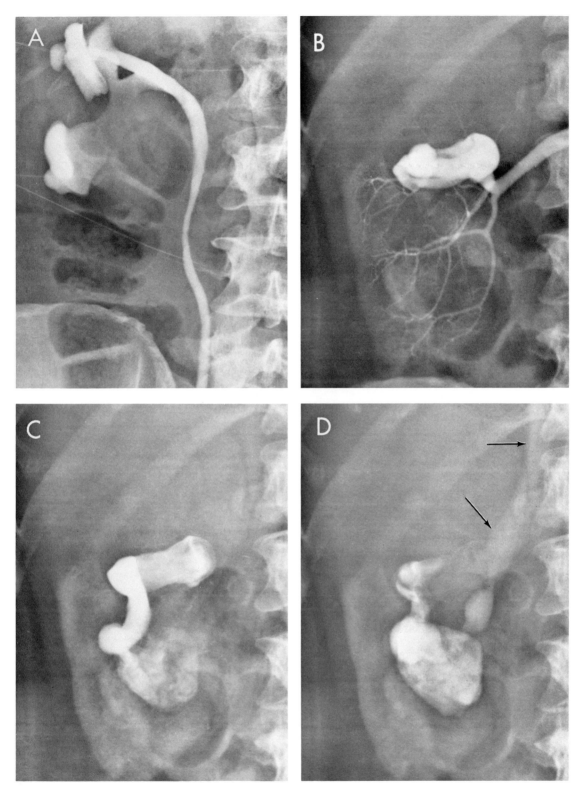

Figure 107 · Arteriovenous Malformation / 331

Figure 108.—Pseudotumor due to an intrarenal hematoma.

A, intravenous urogram, anteroposterior projection: Clearly demonstrating a mass displacing the middle and lower pole calyces of the right kidney (**x**). The mass appears lucent in comparison to the nephrogram in the remaining portions of the kidney.

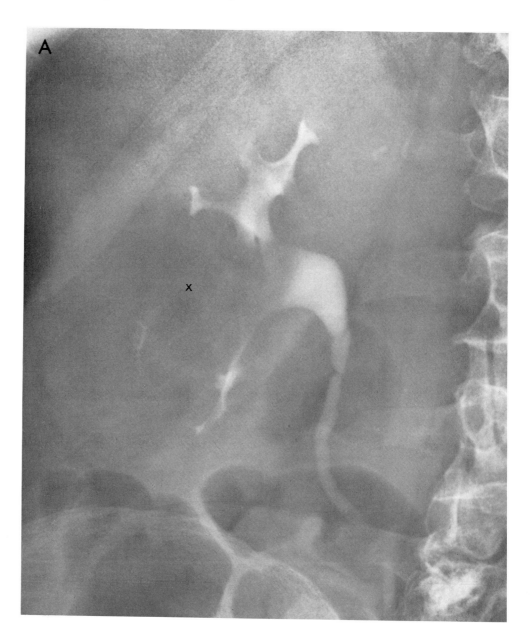

B, nephrotomogram, anteroposterior projection: Demonstrating a large, somewhat uneven radiolucent mass in the middle and lower portions of the right kidney (**arrows**). The margins of the mass are poorly defined and lack the sharp interface with the adjacent opacified parenchyma usually present with simple benign cysts.

(*Continued* on p. 334.)

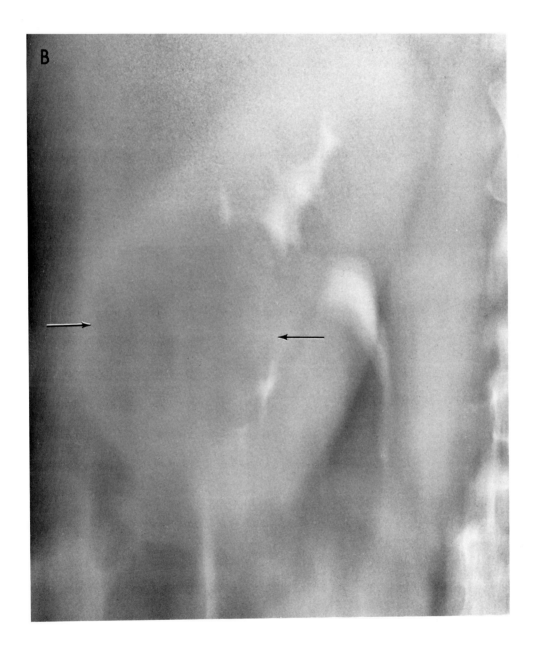

Figure 108 · Intrarenal Hematoma / 333

Figure 108 (cont.).—Pseudotumor due to an intrarenal hematoma.

C, intravenous urogram 11 days after **A** and **B,** anteroposterior exposure: Showing that the mass has disappeared and the collecting system now appears to be normal.

A 53-year-old man was hospitalized because of right flank pain. He was receiving anticoagulation therapy. Because of the history of anticoagulation therapy it was decided that the renal mass was an intrarenal hematoma and the treatment was stopped. The pain abated and in 11 days the hematoma was shown to have resorbed.

Comment: Recognition by physicians of this potential complication of anticoagulation therapy is obviously of extreme importance so that exploratory surgery will not be performed in this type of case, particularly since radiographic studies in some instances may not be able to distinguish this lesion from a renal neoplasm. Intrarenal hematomas are most often caused by anticoagulation therapy and trauma but also are seen in patients with blood dyscrasias, hemorrhagic infarcts, bleeding neoplasms and rupture of an intrarenal artery aneurysm. If an intrarenal hematoma can be suspected from the clinical history, follow-up intravenous urography in about two weeks should show disappearance or decrease of the size of the mass, thereby negating the need for further diagnostic investigation or surgery (see Navani *et al.* below).

Figure 108, courtesy of Dr. P. A. McLellan; from Navani, S.; Bosniak, M. A.; Shapiro, J. H., and Kaufman, S.: Varied radiographic manifestations of urinary tract bleeding, J. Urol. 100:339, 1968.

C

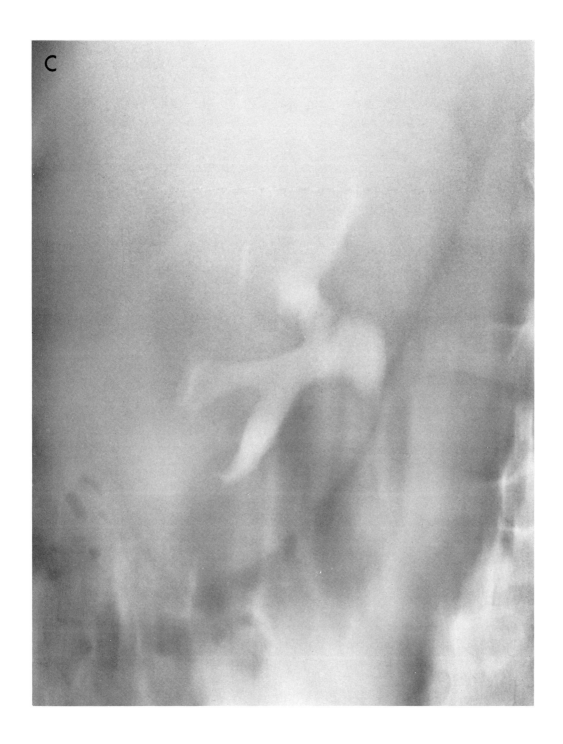

Figure 108 · Intrarenal Hematoma / 335

PART 7

Tumors and Pseudotumors of the Renal Pelvis

Clinical Aspects of Carcinoma
of the Renal Pelvis

CARCINOMA of the renal pelvis represents approximately 8–10% of all malignancies of the kidney. Most of them are transitional cell carcinomas, but occasionally squamous cell carcinomas and rarely adenocarcinomas are also observed.

TRANSITIONAL CELL CARCINOMA

From 80–85% of carcinomas of the renal pelvis are papillary type transitional cell carcinomas. The majority of them are noninfiltrating papillary tumors, although some papillary tumors infiltrate into muscle and the surrounding structures. Transitional cell papillomas are reported in the literature, but these are usually grouped with carcinomas, and for practical purposes every papillary tumor that is clinically recognized should be considered to be carcinoma.

Transitional cell tumors are usually solitary, although they may be bilateral (Fig. 117). Associated tumors have been noted in the distal ureter and in the bladder in 25–50% of reported cases; these are thought to represent metastases from the pelvic tumor, although the concept of a multicentric origin is considered by many authorities. The tumors may arise in a calyx or infundibulum (Fig. 113) but most often occur in the renal pelvis. Patients with these tumors often complain of hematuria as the only clinical symptom, but flank pain due to obstruction and hydronephrosis is not uncommon. Transitional cell carcinoma is more common in men than in women (3:1) and is usually seen in patients over 60 years of age. Renal pelvic tumors spread by direct extension, involving the renal vein in 40–50% of cases, and metastasize usually to lungs, liver, lymph nodes and bones.

SQUAMOUS CELL CARCINOMA

Approximately 15–20% of tumors of the renal pelvis are squamous cell carcinomas. These tumors are almost always associated with long-standing chronic infection and calculous disease. Leukoplakia is considered to be a precursor of this type of neoplasm. Squamous cell carcinomas of the renal pelvis are flat, nonpapillary infiltrating lesions that are more invasive than the transitional cell variety and the prognosis is much worse. Metastases are often present at the time diagnosis is made. There is equal distribution in men and women, and the mean age of patients with this tumor is 55 years.

Squamous cell carcinomas spread by direct extension into the wall of the renal pelvis and down the ureter, and not infrequently they extend into the kidney cortex, amputating and encasing the renal vasculature and calyceal structures (Figs. 120 and 121). The prognosis of these tumors is considered to be worse than that of the transitional cell variety because of their invasive characteristics and because of their more insidious onset which is possibly masked by the coexisting renal calculous or inflammatory disease.

ADENOCARCINOMA

This is an extremely rare tumor of the renal pelvis which represents either a tumor in a congenital tissue malformation or more likely "a further manifestation of the metaplastic changes initiated by chronic irritation or inflammation or both" (Lucké and Schlumberger).

BIBLIOGRAPHY

Emmett, J. L.: *Clinical Urography* (2nd ed.; Philadelphia: W. B. Saunders Company, 1964).

Lucké, B., and Schlumberger, H. G.: "Tumors of the Kidney, Renal Pelvis and Ureter"; Sec. VIII, Fasc. 30 of Armed Forces Institute of Pathology *Atlas of Tumor Pathology* (Washington, D.C., 1957).

Riches, E. (ed.): *Tumours of the Kidney and Ureter* (Baltimore: Williams & Wilkins Company, 1964).

Figure 109.—Leukoplakia.

Intravenous urogram, anteroposterior projection: Revealing a filling defect in the lower pole calyx and infundibulum of the right kidney (**arrow**). Note the somewhat linear striated appearance of the defect. The collecting system is otherwise intact and normal in appearance.

A 65-year-old man was hospitalized with urinary tract infection. He underwent right renal exploration and nephrectomy was performed. The pathologic diagnosis indicated leukoplakia of the renal pelvis and the lower pole calyx.

Comment: Leukoplakia is squamous metaplasia of the transitional epithelium that lines the renal pelvis. It is considered to be a precursor of squamous cell carcinoma and is usually treated by nephrectomy if unilateral. The condition is usually associated with long-standing chronic irritation (calculi) and inflammation. Radiologically the condition cannot be clearly separated from renal pelvic neoplasm and presents the picture of an irregular filling defect in the collecting system. Cholesteatoma is another example of squamous metaplasia of the epithelial lining and is a progressive stage of leukoplakia. Radiologically it is indistinguishable from the filling defects of leukoplakia and renal pelvic carcinoma.*

---

* Noyes, W. E., and Palubinskas, A. J.: Squamous metaplasia of the renal pelvis, Radiology 89:292, 1967.

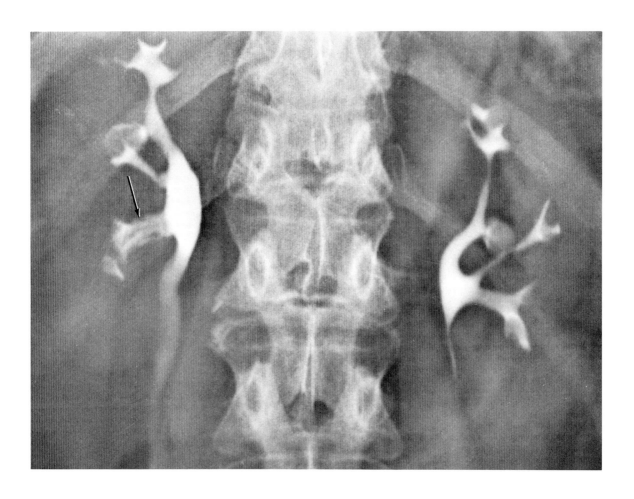

Figure 109 · Leukoplakia / 341

Figure 110.—Leukoplakia.

Left retrograde pyelogram, anteroposterior projection: Showing small filling defects involving the renal pelvis and upper ureter (**arrows**). The calyces show good cupping and no evidence of pyelonephritis.

A man of 52 was hospitalized because of micturition every one to two hours day and night. He also complained of suprapubic pain and passage of "tissue" per urethra. An intravenous urogram revealed irregular filling of both renal pelves, more pronounced on the left. He underwent left renal exploration. Biopsy examination of tissue from the wall of the renal pelvis revealed squamous metaplasia (leukoplakia).

Comment: Irregular small filling defects of this nature should suggest the possibility of leukoplakia. The same type of defect might, however, represent transitional cell carcinoma or ureteritis and pyelitis cystica. The last would be less likely in this case since no evidence of pyelonephritis is apparent in the kidney and the defects are somewhat more irregular than the round cystlike lesions of pyelitis cystica. Angiography was performed, with negative results, as would be expected. The surgeon chose not to perform a nephrectomy, even though the condition is considered to be premalignant, because both kidneys were involved by the process.

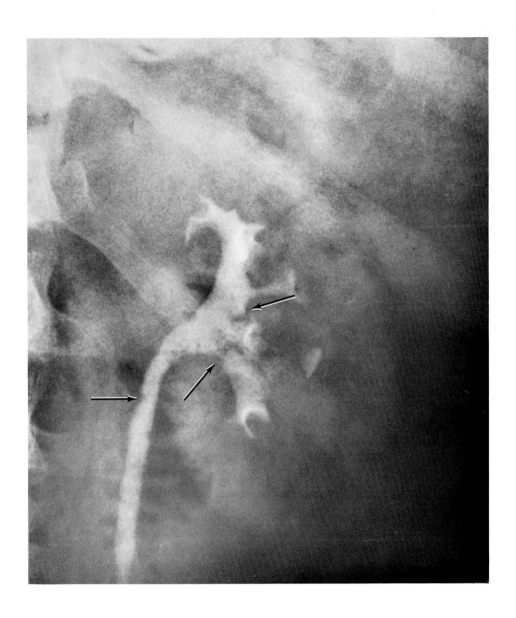

Figure 110 · Leukoplakia / 343

Figure 111.—Papillary transitional cell carcinoma of the renal pelvis.

A, right retrograde pyelogram, anteroposterior projection: Showing a ragged destructive lesion involving the entire upper pole calyx and extending into the renal pelvis.

B, surgical specimen: Showing a 3×4 cm tumor (**arrows**) extending along the superior margin of the renal pelvis.

A man of 60 was hospitalized because of recurrent hematuria. Intravenous urography revealed irregularity of the upper pole calyx of the right kidney. Right nephroureterectomy was performed for papillary transitional cell carcinoma. Four months later he was rehospitalized because of hematuria. Cystoscopy revealed multiple small (0.5–1.0 cm) papillary lesions at the bladder base, proved to represent transitional cell carcinoma of the bladder.

Comment: The urographic appearance of this lesion is characteristic of carcinoma of the renal pelvis and infundibulum. Inflammatory disease would not be expected to cause the type of filling defects and irregularity seen in this case. Selective right renal angiography revealed no definite abnormality. Negative results of angiography in pelvic lesions do not rule out malignancy; with these tumors arteriography is not as important as pyelography. Angiography should be performed, however, because preoperative demonstration of the renal anatomy aids the surgeon in planning nephrectomy and because occasionally tumor vessels are seen which further confirms the preoperative diagnosis.

This case also illustrates a common clinical pattern in these patients—recurrent hematuria due to metastatic foci in the bladder. Patients who present multiple bladder lesions should be carefully and thoroughly evaluated for possible lesions of the renal pelvis.

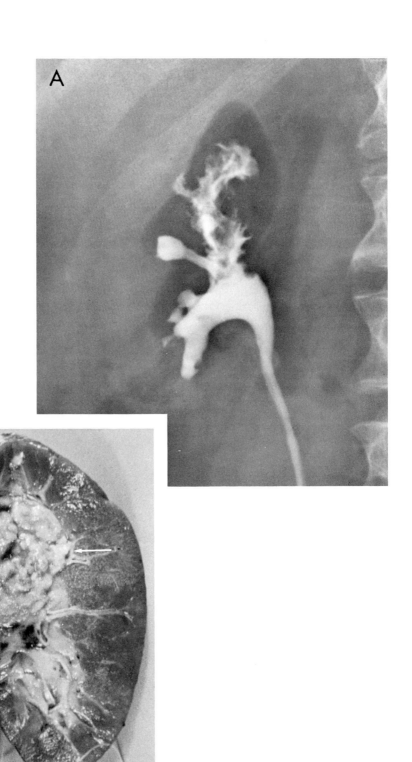

Figure 111 · Transitional Cell Carcinoma / 345

Figure 112.—Papillary transitional cell carcinoma of the renal pelvis.

Left retrograde pyelogram, anteroposterior projection: Showing a large irregular filling defect occupying the left renal pelvis. The defect in the inferior margin of the pelvis (**arrow**) represents the site of tumor attachment.

A 62-year-old woman entered the hospital because of hematuria. An intravenous pyelogram revealed a filling defect in the left renal pelvis. Left ureteronephrectomy was performed for papillary transitional cell carcinoma of the renal pelvis.

Comment: This is the classic pyelographic appearance of a large papillary type of renal pelvic carcinoma. The diagnosis of stone and blood clot can be ruled out by demonstrating that the lesion does not move with changes of position of the patient and also because of the irregular contour of the renal pelvis at the site of attachment with the lesion.

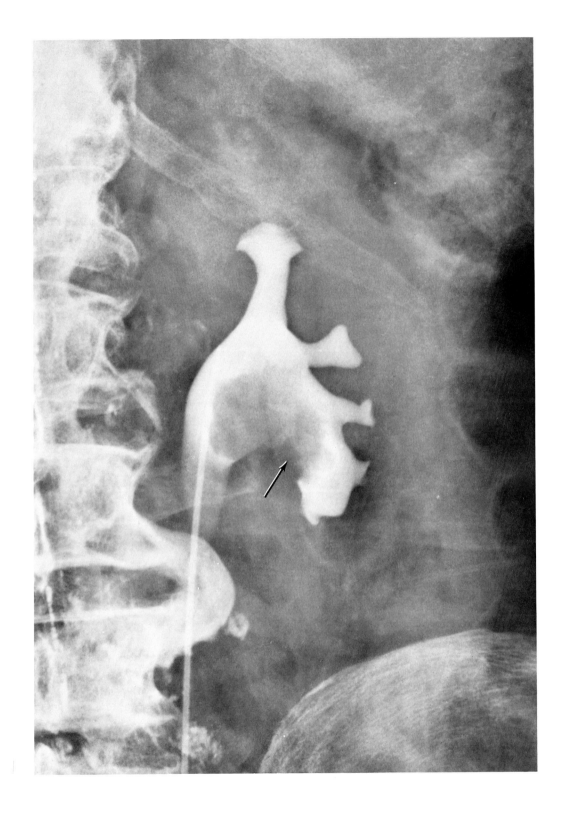

Figure 112 · Transitional Cell Carcinoma / 347

Figure 113.—Papillary carcinoma of the upper pole infundibulum.

A, intravenous urogram, anteroposterior projection: Indicating amputation of the upper pole calyx (**arrow**) and indistinct outline of the left kidney.

B, retrograde pyelogram, anteroposterior exposure: Demonstrating irregular cavitarylike defect (**arrow**) producing obstruction of the upper pole calyx.

A 51-year-old man was asymptomatic until two months before examination, when he had a shaking chill followed by fever. He was hospitalized for diagnostic study. At surgery a papillary carcinoma of the infundibulum was found.

Comment: In the intravenous urogram, the failure of visualization of the upper pole calyx could be due to neoplasm, inflammation (particularly tuberculosis) or stone. In the retrograde pyelogram, a similar filling defect deformity might be caused by a radiolucent stone, blood clot, crossing vessel or proteinaceous cast. Angiography in the presence of a small papillary lesion of this type often fails to delineate tumor vasculature and therefore may not be helpful. However, it should be performed to rule out the possibility that the defect in the infundibulum is due to pressure by an overlying vessel (Fig. 122) and to evaluate the total extent of the tumor (Fig. 121). Clinical evaluation might be able to differentiate these possibilities, but usually exploratory surgery is needed.

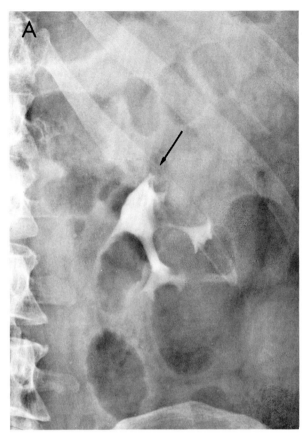

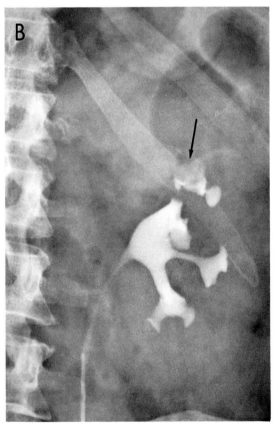

Figure 113 · Papillary Carcinoma / 349

Figure 114.—Transitional cell carcinoma of the renal pelvis with progression over a three month period.

A, intravenous urogram, anteroposterior projection: Showing a large discrete filling defect occupying the central portion of the right renal pelvis (**x**). There are also numerous smaller, less well defined filling defects extending into the proximal ureter.

B, intravenous urogram, three months after **A,** anteroposterior view: Indicating that a pronounced change has taken place in the interval. The entire pelvis has a ragged disrupted appearance with irregular borders accompanied by obstructive caliectasis. Some of the filling defects may also represent associated blood clots.

A man of 68 was hospitalized because of symptoms of prostatism and hematuria of four weeks' duration. He underwent prostatectomy but continued to have hematuria and returned three months later for further study (**B**). Right nephroureterectomy was performed for a papillary type transitional carcinoma of the renal pelvis. In the following three years the patient was seen in the hospital seven times for fulguration of recurrent bladder tumors.

Comment: This case gives us the opportunity to see the radiographic progression of a transitional cell carcinoma of the renal pelvis over a three month period. Recurrent bladder tumors are commonly associated with these lesions; it is not clear whether this is due to seeding from the original lesion or represents multicentric foci of tumor.

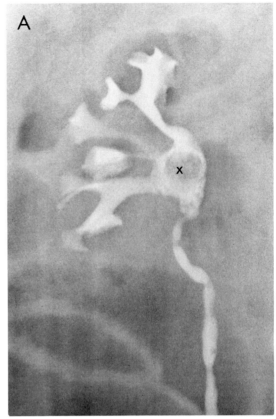

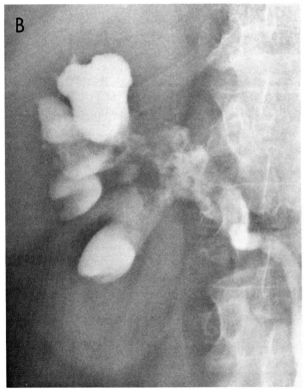

Figure 114 · Transitional Cell Carcinoma / 351

Figure 115.—Transitional cell carcinoma of the renal pelvis with extension down the ureter and hydronephrosis; angiography.

A, selective right renal arteriogram, arterial phase, anteroposterior projection: Showing typical changes of hydronephrosis with stretching of the intrarenal branches over dilated calyceal structures. A hypertrophied pelvic artery (**arrow**), a branch of the renal artery, gives off a cluster of tumorlike vessels to the renal pelvis (**a**) and continues down along the ureter supplying the ureteral extension of the tumor (**b**).

(*Continued* on p. 354.)

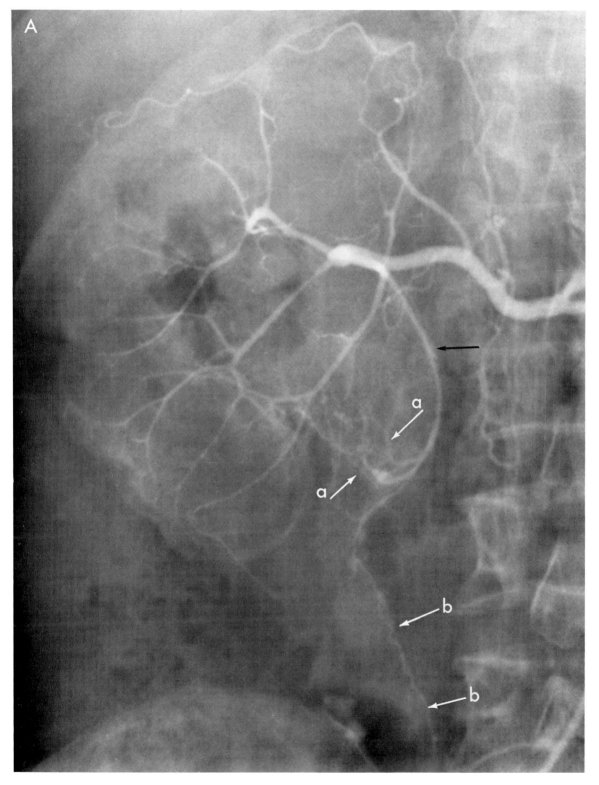

Figure 115 · Transitional Cell Carcinoma / 353

Figure 115 (cont.).—Transitional cell carcinoma of the renal pelvis with extension down the ureter and hydronephrosis; angiography.

B, same study as **A,** nephrogram phase: Demonstrating the shell of a hydronephrotic kidney. The outline of the tumor in the renal pelvis and upper ureter can be identified from the slight blush of tumor tissue in these areas (**arrows**).

C, surgical specimen: Revealing transitional cell carcinoma filling the renal pelvis and upper ureter. Hydronephrosis of the kidney is present.

A man of 65 was hospitalized because of hematuria. An intravenous urogram revealed no function of the right kidney. Retrograde pyelography could not be performed because of an enlarged prostate. Right nephrectomy and ureterectomy were performed.

Comment: This is an example of an occasional presentation of renal pelvic carcinoma—nonvisualization of the kidney on urography owing to hydronephrosis. Usually retrograde pyelography is then performed, which elucidates the problem. Occasionally, however, retrograde pyelography cannot be accomplished, as in this case, or fails to demonstrate the cause of obstruction. In such instances angiography can be diagnostic and clearly define the pathology,* as illustrated here.

---

* Boijsen, E., and Folin, J.: Angiography in carcinoma of the renal pelvis, Acta radiol. 56:81, 1961.

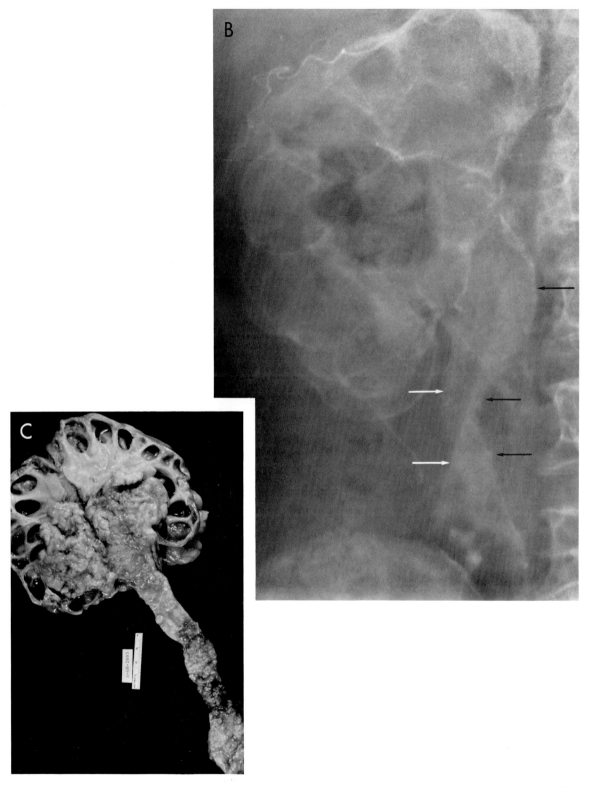

Figure 115 · Transitional Cell Carcinoma / 355

Figure 116.—Papillary transitional cell carcinoma of the renal pelvis.

A, left retrograde pyelogram with patient supine, anteroposterior projection: Delineating a lobulated filling defect in the renal pelvis (**x**).

B, same study with the patient erect: Showing the lobulated defect in the same position in the renal pelvis as in **A,** indicating that it is attached to the wall and is not freely movable in the pelvis.

A 45-year-old man had had repeated episodes of painless gross hematuria at intervals for a year before hospitalization. An intravenous urogram revealed a filling defect in the left renal pelvis. On left nephrectomy a transitional cell carcinoma was found. The tumor measured $1.5 \times 1.2 \times 1.4$ cm and was lobulated and pedunculated.

Comment: The radiographic findings in this case are quite characteristic of papillary type transitional cell carcinoma. A blood clot or calculus might give this appearance on the pyelogram, but the failure of the defect to change position when the patient's position is changed from supine to erect indicates that the lesion is attached to the pelvic wall, suggesting a neoplasm. Also, the lobulated, irregular borders suggest that neoplasm is the likely diagnosis.

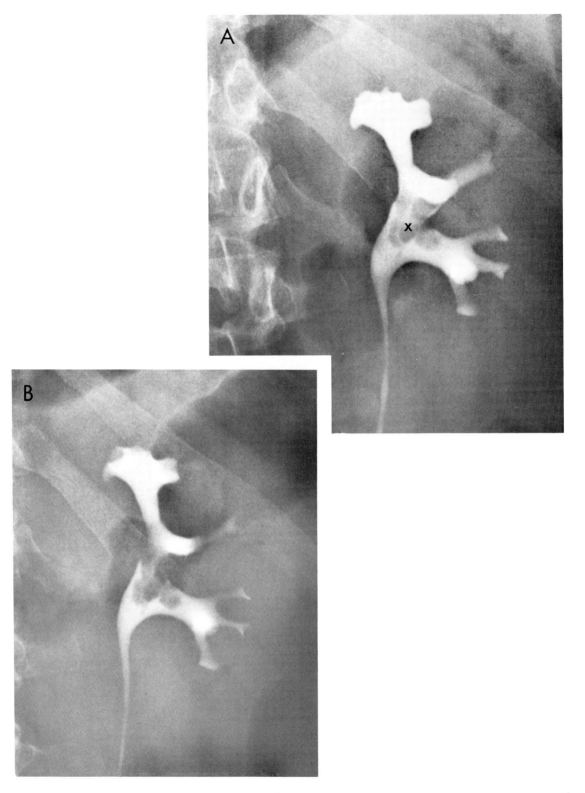

Figure 116 · Papillary Carcinoma / 357

Figure 117.—Bilateral papillary type carcinomas of the renal pelves.

Bilateral retrograde pyelogram, anteroposterior projection: Revealing a round sharply defined radiolucent filling defect 1 cm in diameter in the upper portion of the right renal pelvis (**a**) and a small (4–5 mm) round radiolucent defect in the left renal pelvis (**b**).

A man of 52 entered the hospital for follow-up evaluation. He had recurrent bladder tumors that had required multiple transurethral resections of the bladder over a 10 year period. An intravenous urogram revealed a filling defect in the right renal pelvis. He underwent a partial right nephrectomy for a papillary type transitional cell carcinoma of the right renal pelvis. Later he had a left pyelotomy for excision of the lesion of the left renal pelvis which proved to be a well-differentiated papilloma (low-grade papillary carcinoma).

Comment: This is an unusual case of bilateral renal pelvis carcinomas in association with multiple bladder carcinomas. Similar cases have been reported. This case supports the concept of multicentric origin of these tumors. Usually, however, when multiple papillary tumors are found in the renal pelvis, the ipsilateral ureter and ipsilateral part of the bladder are affected.*

---

* Emmett, J. L.: *Clinical Urography* (2nd ed.; Philadelphia: W. B. Saunders Company, 1964).

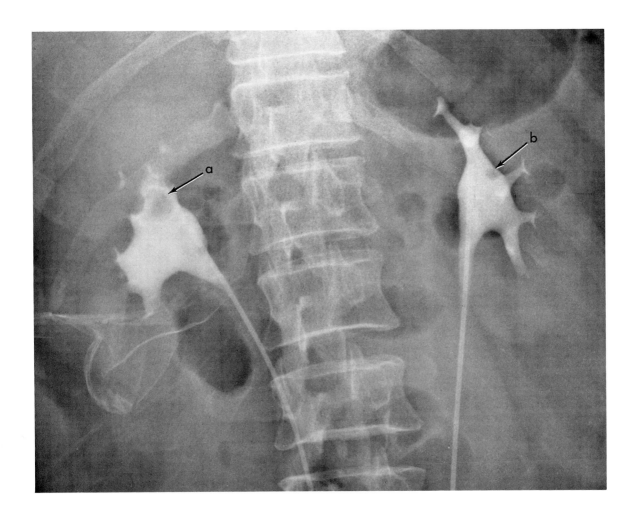

Figure 117 · Bilateral Papillary Carcinoma / 359

Figure 118.—Transitional cell carcinoma of the renal pelvis.

A, left retrograde pyelogram, anteroposterior exposure: Showing irregular filling defects involving the renal pelvis with extensive destruction of renal parenchyma and calyces.

B, selective left renal arteriogram, late arterial phase, anteroposterior view: Demonstrating irregular, beaded and tortuous vessels in the superior portion of the renal hilus and upper pole (**arrows**). These are typical neoplastic vessels.

A man of 59 was hospitalized because of hematuria. A left nephrectomy was performed. Pathologic diagnosis was papillary transitional cell carcinoma of the renal pelvis with invasion of the kidney, secondary atrophy and chronic inflammation.

Comment: In this case the diagnosis of carcinoma of the renal pelvis is mainly made by the pyelographic appearance of the lesion, while angiography confirms the diagnosis and nicely demonstrates the extent of the tumor. Small noninfiltrating papillary tumors usually do not contain abnormal blood vessels. Infiltrating tumors do reveal such abnormalities, showing either "abnormal" vessels (Fig. 119) or encasement and amputation of vessels (Fig. 121). Unfortunately, the latter angiographic picture may occasionally be seen in chronic inflammatory disease, which therefore limits the diagnostic role of angiography in some of these lesions.*

---

* Watson, R., and Fleming, R. J.: Tumors and Infections of the Renal Pelvis: Role of Arteriography in Diagnosis. Paper presented at the annual meeting of the Radiological Society of North America, December, 1969.

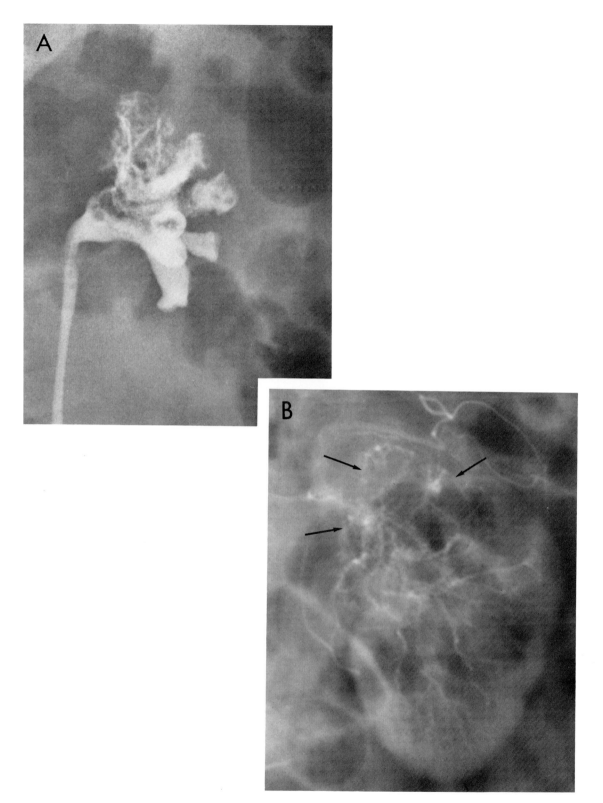

Figure 118 · Transitional Cell Carcinoma / 361

Figure 119.—Papillary carcinoma of the renal pelvis.

A, intravenous urogram, anteroposterior exposure: Showing hydrone-phrotic changes in the left kidney. The renal pelvis is only partially filled and has irregular filling defects and shaggy border (**arrow**).

B, retrograde pyelogram, anteroposterior view: Revealing multiple irregular filling defects involving the renal pelvis and upper ureter and extending into the lower pole infundibulum and calyces. The shaggy borders and ragged, moth-eaten appearance are characteristic of neoplasm of the renal pelvis.

C, selective left renal arteriogram, anteroposterior view: Demonstrating numerous abnormal-appearing vessels in the region of the renal pelvis and extending into the cortex of the kidney in the middle and lower poles (**a**). Note hypertrophy of pelvic and ureteral vessels feeding the neoplasm (**b**).

A 67-year-old woman was examined because of painless hematuria. A left nephrectomy and ureterectomy were performed. The pathologic diagnosis was papillary carcinoma arising from the renal pelvis and extending superficially into the lower pole of the kidney.

Comment: The role of angiography in the diagnosis of renal pelvic tumors will vary with the type of tumor and its pyelographic appearance. For instance, in Figure 111 the diagnosis of a tumor of the renal pelvis was made entirely on the basis of the pyelogram; the angiogram showed no definite abnormality. However, in Figure 115, the diagnosis was made by angiography, as pyelography could not be performed. Likewise in Figure 121, the diagnosis is unclear on pyelography but is diagnostic of renal pelvic carcinoma on angiography. In other instances the pyelogram might indicate carcinoma and the angiogram will corroborate the diagnosis, as in this case and in Figure 118. Occasionally, utilizing routine pyelography, it is difficult to distinguish between a parenchymal tumor with invasion of the collecting system and a primary collecting system lesion with extension into the parenchyma. Angiography is usually able to make the differentiation. This is of more than academic interest since the treatment for renal pelvic carcinoma is generally total nephroureterectomy while for renal cell carcinoma it is nephrectomy alone.

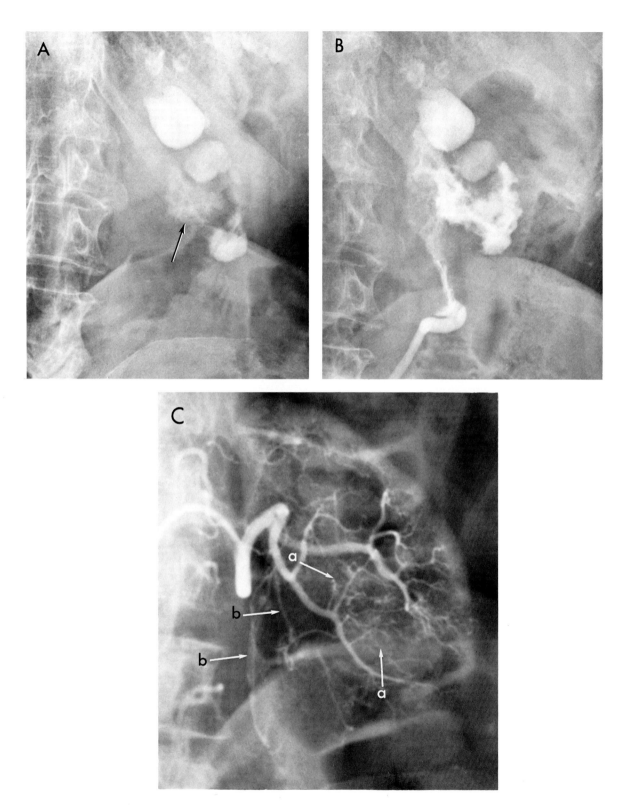

Figure 119 · Papillary Carcinoma / 363

Figure 120.—Squamous cell carcinoma of the renal pelvis extending into the renal cortex.

A, chest film, posteroanterior projection: Revealing a large density in the left lung and multiple small round densities throughout both lung fields indicative of metastatic carcinoma.

B, right retrograde pyelogram, anteroposterior exposure: With contrast medium outlining a mass (**arrows**) which occupies and occludes the renal pelvis.

C, selective right renal arteriogram, arterial phase, anteroposterior view: Demonstrating poor filling of vessels in the upper pole which are attenuated but not displaced (**a**). The capsular artery courses above the upper pole (**b**). Note irregular tortuous vessels in the region of the renal pelvis (**c**). Vessels in the rest of the kidney are essentially normal.

(*Continued* on p. 366.)

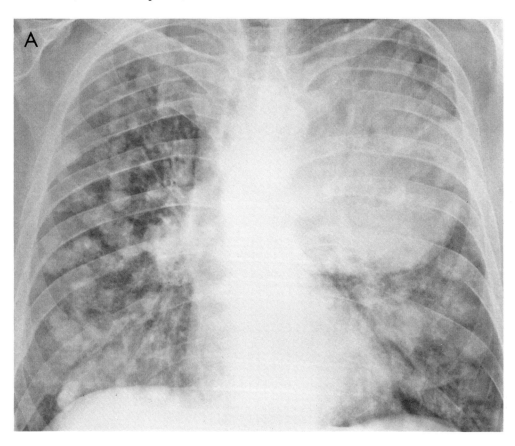

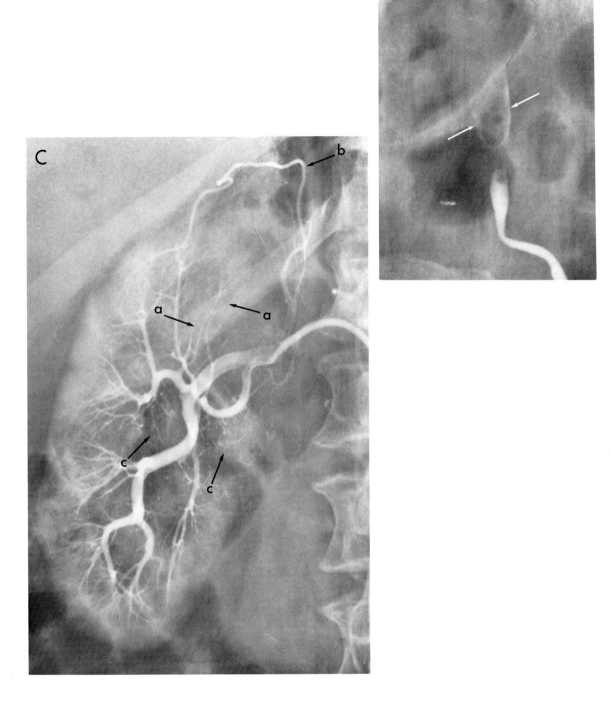

Figure 120 · Squamous Cell Carcinoma / 365

Figure 120 (cont.).—Squamous cell carcinoma of the renal pelvis extending into the renal cortex.

D, same study, nephrogram phase: Revealing a distinctly diminished nephrogram in the upper portion of the kidney. There is stasis of contrast medium in small tortuous vessels in the renal pelvis (**arrow**).

E, autopsy specimen of right kidney, three months after radiographic studies: Showing replacement of the upper and middle poles of the kidney by tumor. There is also tumor in the hilus (**arrow**). Only in the lower pole is normal renal tissue present. The specimen shows more extensive involvement by neoplasm than does the angiogram (**C** and **D**) because three months had elapsed since angiography.

A man of 61 had gross painless hematuria. On intravenous urography the right kidney was not visualized. A percutaneous lung biopsy specimen revealed undifferentiated epidermoid carcinoma. Three months later he died of widely disseminated disease. At autopsy, tumor was found in both kidneys, adrenal and lungs. Histologically it was squamous cell carcinoma.

Comment: The pathologist could not decide whether this was a squamous cell carcinoma of the renal pelvis extending into the cortex and metastasizing into the other kidney, adrenals and lungs or a carcinoma of the lung with metastases to the aforementioned areas. Renal angiography in both instances would give a similar picture, but the tumor vessels in the area of the renal pelvis and the filling defect in the renal pelvis noted in the retrograde pyelogram suggests that the tumor originated in the renal pelvis. Attenuation of vessels, encasement, amputation and diminished nephrogram without displacement of vessels is typical of neoplasms which infiltrate the renal cortex as seen with carcinoma of the renal pelvis when it infiltrates into the renal cortex, metastatic squamous cell carcinoma to the kidney (Fig. 85) and occasionally lymphoma (Fig. 87).

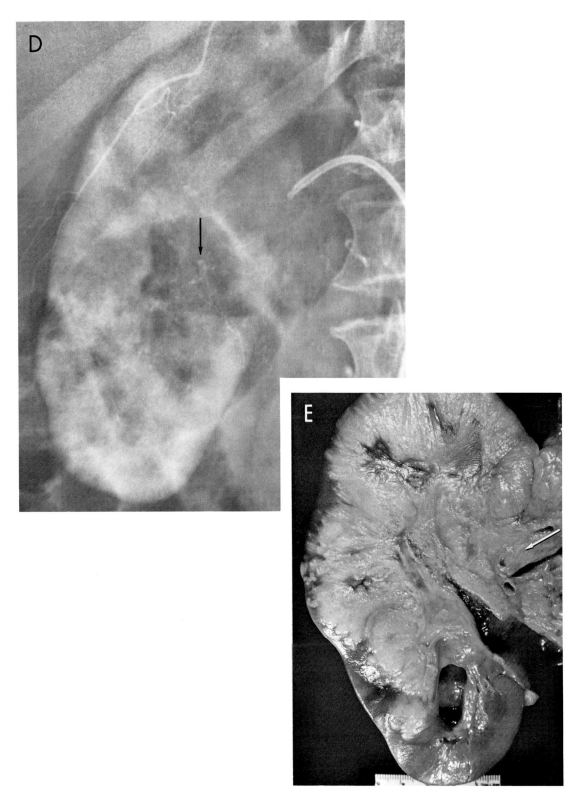

Figure 120 · Squamous Cell Carcinoma / 367

Figure 121.—Squamous cell carcinoma of the renal pelvis with invasion of the renal parenchyma.

A, intravenous urogram, anteroposterior projection: Failing to demonstrate the upper pole infundibulum and calyx of the right kidney. The contour of the upper pole appears to be normal. There are small irregular filling defects in the renal pelvis.

B, selective right renal arteriogram, anteroposterior view: Showing a decrease in number of vessels in the upper pole of the kidney and diminished intensity of the nephrogram in this area. Some vessels are amputated and irregular due to tumor encasement (**a**). Hypertrophy and tortuosity of pelvic and ureteral arteries (**b**) are also present.

A man of 62 entered the hospital for follow-up urologic study two years after radical cystectomy for carcinoma of the bladder. An ileal conduit had been constructed at that time. After these radiographic studies a right nephrectomy was performed. A squamous cell carcinoma of the renal pelvis was found, with invasion of the renal parenchyma and ureter.

Comment: This is the typical appearance of an invasive type of tumor. The angiogram shows only a few tumor vessels but definite evidence of tumor extension and encasement.*

---

* Mitty, H. A.; Baron, M. G., and Feller, M.: Infiltrating carcinoma of the renal pelvis: Angiographic features, Radiology 92:994, 1969; Becker, J. A., and Kanter, I. E.: Arterial encasement in transitional cell carcinoma, J. Canad. A. Radiol. 19:203, 1968.

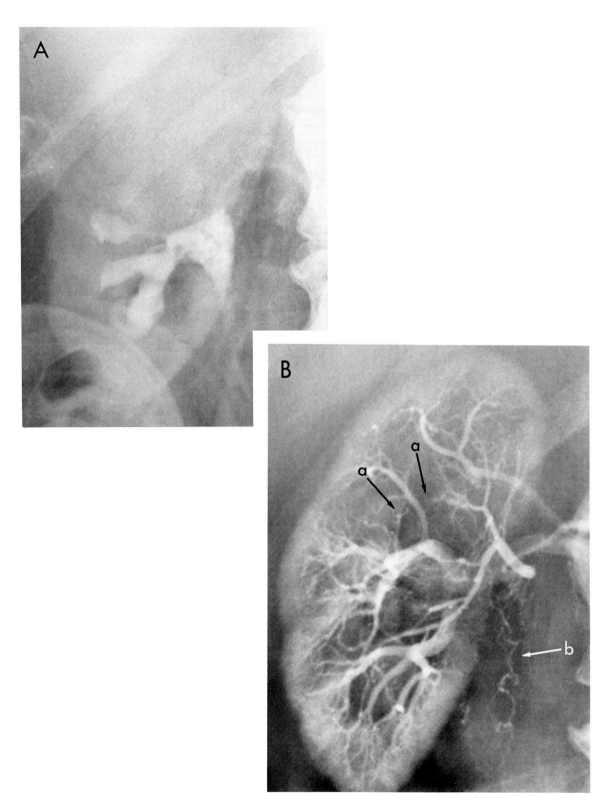

Figure 121 · Squamous Cell Carcinoma / 369

Figure 122.—Pseudotumor of the infundibulum due to pressure by an overlying vessel.

A, left retrograde pyelogram, anteroposterior exposure: Showing a persistent defect in the upper pole infundibulum (**arrow**). There is no evidence of dilatation of the upper pole calyces.

B, selective left renal arteriogram, anteroposterior exposure: Showing that the main branch of the left renal artery crosses and indents the upper pole infundibulum (**arrows**).

A 63-year-old man was hospitalized because of fever and pyuria. An intravenous urogram revealed incomplete filling of the upper pole infundibulum of the left kidney.

Comment: Impressions by vessels on the renal collecting systems are common and usually show a characteristic picture. The area most often affected is the infundibulum to the upper pole, as in this case. Ocassionally angiography is needed to establish the diagnosis and rule out a pelvic tumor.*

---

* Kreel, L., and Pyle, R.: Arterial impressions of the renal pelvis, Brit. J. Radiol. 35:609, 1962.

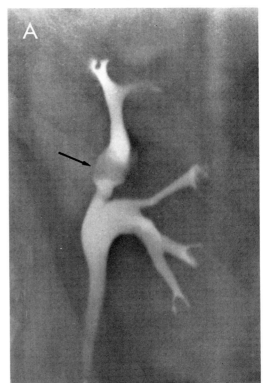

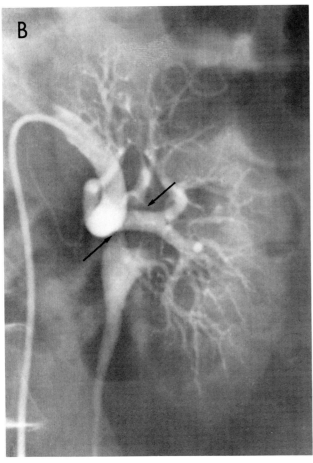

Figure 122 · Pseudotumor / 371

Figure 123.—Blood clot in the renal pelvis simulating renal tumor.

Right retrograde pyelogram, anteroposterior projection: Showing irregular filling defects in the right renal pelvis.

A 62-year-old man underwent a right ureterolithotomy for a right ureteral calculus. Four days later he had right renal colic. An intravenous urogram revealed nonvisualization of the right collecting system with a nephrogram on the late film. After right retrograde pyelography (shown here) blood clots were irrigated and the catheter then drained well. A week later a repeat intravenous urogram was normal.

Comment: The filling defect in the renal pelvis caused by a blood clot may be indistinguishable from a papillary tumor. In the case illustrated here the diagnosis was obvious from the history of recent surgery in the area. Occasionally, however, in a patient with gross hematuria and presenting a filling defect in the renal pelvis the differentiation between blood clot and tumor may be quite difficult. Both may have irregular contours, but blood clots occasionally present as casts of infundibular structures and also change shape and position with changes of body position. If blood clot is suspected, irrigation of the renal pelvis and repeat urography are indicated.

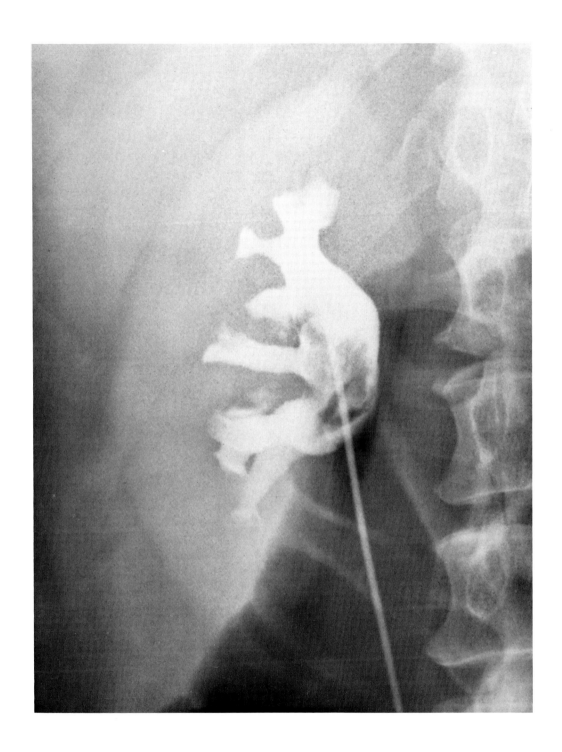

Figure 123 · Pseudotumor / 373

Figure 124.—Pseudotumor due to a uric acid calculus.

Retrograde pyelogram, anteroposterior projection: Demonstrating a well-defined ovoid filling defect in the renal pelvis, the margins of which are sharp and smooth.

A 67-year-old man was hospitalized because of left flank pain. He had a history of uric acid calculus. An intravenous urogram revealed hydronephrosis of the left kidney and evidence of obstruction at the ureteropelvic junction.

Comment: This is an instance in which retrograde pyelography is needed for optimal demonstration of a renal pelvis filling defect. On the basis of the pyelogram, the principal diagnostic considerations are tumor, stone and blood clot. The very sharp, smooth and well-marginated outlines of the defect favor diagnosis of a benign lesion but by no means exclude the possibility of a malignant tumor. The history in this case of a uric acid calculus is important. A left pyelolithotomy removed a 1×3 cm stone impacted at the ureteropelvic junction.

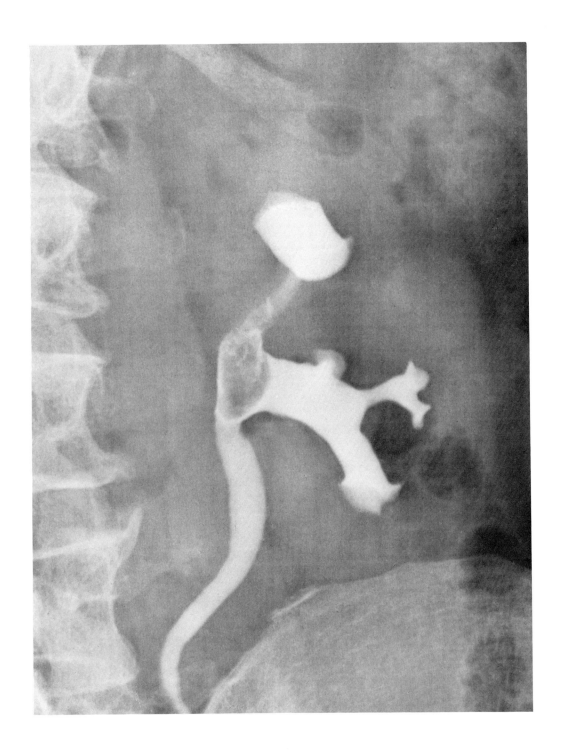

Figure 124 · Pseudotumor / 375

Index